PATIENT-
CENTRED
CONSULTING
FOR THE
MRCGP

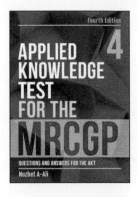
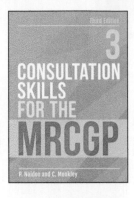
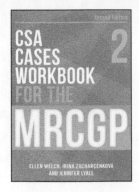
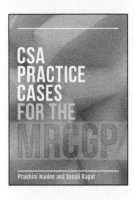
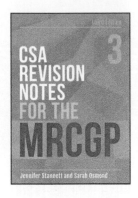
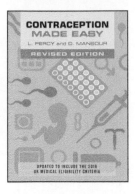
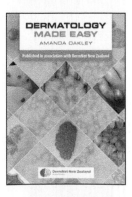
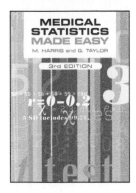
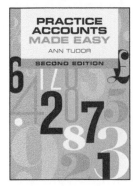

PATIENT-CENTRED CONSULTING FOR THE MRCGP

Chinedu Odina MBBS, MRCGP, DRCOG, DGM
GP Trainer, Southend-on-Sea

Scion

© **Scion Publishing Limited, 2017**

ISBN 978 1 911510 06 2

First published 2017

A CIP catalogue record for this book is available from the British Library.

Scion Publishing Limited

The Old Hayloft, Vantage Business Park, Bloxham Road, Banbury OX16 9UX, UK

www.scionpublishing.com

Important Note from the Publisher

Typeset by Medlar Publishing Solutions Pvt Ltd, India

Printed in the UK

Contents

Contents

Preface

The CSA examination assesses the ability of the doctor to gather information, apply learned understanding of disease processes, make shared decisions and communicate effectively with patients.[1] The task in the structured setting of the examination is to integrate these skills effectively. To achieve this level of integration, doctors would normally have practised these skills as recommended in the competency framework to flexibly integrate the skills in consultations effectively. Developing the skills required to achieve an effective consultation can be challenging without repeated reflection on performance by self or peer, using an accurate understanding of the meaning of the competencies. This understanding is normally facilitated by trainers. This book was written to augment the efforts of trainees and trainers in self/peer assessment using an approach which explores the applicable meaning of the competencies assessed in the CSA, and reflects on the common reasons for failure in the exam.

It is expected that from clinical encounters, reflecting on these experiences and clinical supervision, doctors build their insight and understanding into the meaning of the competencies. This book enhances this transition from unknown unknowns to known unknowns, and assists doctors to identify their strengths/ gaps earlier, facilitating the application and integration of the skills through experiential learning in practice. Doctors early in their training are likely to benefit even more from an earlier appreciation of the meaning of the competencies assessed in the CSA as they are applied in consultations through detailed analysis of doctor/patient dialogues, thus improving the quality of their self-reflections.

In this book, I have used real-life type dialogues to explore the competencies as assessed in the CSA to demonstrate why doctors continue to prepare for the examination with the wrong understanding of the skill level assessed. The dialogues and the analysis in this book focus on the meaning of the competencies assessed in the CSA. The doctor understands the application of the skills and the nature of flexibility and fluency assessed in the CSA to improve their self-reflection from day-to-day patient encounters. The most effective way to master the integration of these skills flexibly and efficiently in consultations is by proactively and routinely applying the right approach in day-to-day encounters. Role plays and simulations have limitations as they are not robust enough to recreate all the components of a real-life encounter.[2]

Using the insight from this book, the approach for the preparation of the CSA will shift from formulaic problem-based rehearsals to patient-centred preparation, rehearsing the competencies required to achieve patient-centredness in any case presentation, independent of the nature of the clinical problem presented. Doctors learning from this book are more likely to enhance their individual styles, applying the insight gained from the book in practice rather than the often-seen instructional case-centred books which distract from the patient-centredness approach of the CSA, creating formulaic habits.

This book is designed to address the common reasons for failure in the CSA examination as published by the RCGP. The CSA assesses the doctor's ability to focus their knowledge of common conditions to the individual patient's experience, using their understanding of the uniqueness of the patient. This book is a guide to how to understand and practise the communication skills required to consult competently. You will achieve fluency through repeated practice using the insights explored in this book.

Dr C. Odina
April 2017

Dedication

I dedicate this book to Ollie.

Chapter 1

Introduction

Who is this book for?

I wrote this book for doctors preparing for the CSA examination as an insight into the meaning of the RCGP competencies. The book uses detailed and analysed dialogues to explore how the doctor should think, how they should behave, and why they should act in a particular way, to enhance their understanding of the meaning of the competencies as they are applied in a consultation. These dialogues will help you to understand and then demonstrate the fluency and integration required to pass the CSA, as opposed to what to do in a particular disease condition, which some preparatory books suggest and which is not what the CSA assesses. This book augments the doctor's in-house training and encourages self-learning from day-to-day practice rather than learning formulaic habits.

Doctors in ST1 and ST2 can use the insights in this book to improve their understanding of the application of the competency areas assessed throughout their work-based placement assessment, improving the quality of their reflections and self/peer assessments.

Setting the stage

The competencies set by the RCGP demonstrate the required level of skill needed to achieve patient-centredness using a recognisable and structured consultation style.[1] Understanding the meaning of these competencies early in training enhances self-reflection/assessment and improves the use of the work-based assessment tools. It is important to note that the CSA is not just a knowledge test but a test of fluent application of the knowledge to achieve patient-centredness, regardless of the case presented. I have explored the real meaning of the competencies as they should be applied in practice, to help doctors work towards what the CSA assesses, rather than formulaic preparation. A doctor who understands the level of skill required to perform at a competent level is more likely to consolidate the use of these skills in their day-to-day practice.

> Throughout this book, there are four main steps to remember as you read. These steps will help you practise patient-centredness in a timely and fluent manner, using the right understanding of the competency and CSA grade descriptors.
>
> 1. Discover the reason for the patient's attendance by actively encouraging the patient's contribution, and recognise the condition using the knowledge of probability based on prevalence.
> 2. Clarify the clinical diagnosis using focused closed questions and examination guided by the probability of the disease, the patient's perspective, and excluding red flags.

3. Explain the problem to the patient, responding to the patient's understanding of the problem and not simply using non-jargon words.
4. Negotiate the plan by taking into account the views of both the patient and the doctor (a partnership).

The application of these steps is developed from understanding the competencies as described by the RCGP competency descriptors outlined below (all reproduced from the RCGP website www.rcgp.org.uk with permission). These competencies are demonstrated individually in this book using many doctor–patient consultations to explore their meaning and application in practice. A doctor who understands why these competencies are valuable, and uses them in real life to explore the benefits of patient-centredness to achieve efficiency and patient satisfaction, is more likely to become fluent in their application.

Communication and consultation skills

This is about communication with patients, the use of recognised consultation techniques, establishing patient partnership, managing challenging consultations, third-party consultations and the use of interpreters.

Insufficient evidence	Needs further development	Competent	Excellent
	Develops a relationship with the patient, which works, but is focused on the problem rather than the patient.	Explores and responds to the patient's agenda, health beliefs and preferences. Elicits psychological and social information to place the patient's problem in context.	Incorporates the patient's perspective and context when negotiating the management plan.
From the available evidence, the doctor's performance cannot be placed on a higher point of this developmental scale.	Uses a rigid or formulaic approach to achieve the main tasks of the consultation.	Achieves the tasks of the consultation, responding to the preferences of the patient in an efficient manner.	Appropriately uses advanced consultation skills, such as confrontation or catharsis, to achieve better patient outcomes.
	The use of language is technically correct but not well adapted to the needs and characteristics of the patient.	The use of language is fluent and takes into consideration the needs and characteristics of the patient, for instance when talking to children or patients with learning disabilities.	Employs a full range of fluent communication skills, both verbal and non-verbal, including active listening skills.
	Provides explanations that are medically correct but doctor-centred.	Uses the patient's understanding to help improve the explanation offered.	Uses a variety of communication techniques and materials (e.g. written or electronic) to adapt explanations to the needs of the patient.

Insufficient evidence	Needs further development	Competent	Excellent
	Communicates management plans but without negotiating with, or involving, the patient.	Works in partnership with the patient, negotiating a mutually acceptable plan that respects the patient's agenda and preference for involvement.	Whenever possible, adopts plans that respect the patient's autonomy. When there is a difference of opinion the patient's autonomy is respected and a positive relationship is maintained.
	Consults to an acceptable standard but lacks focus and requires longer consulting times.	Consults in an organised and structured way, achieving the main tasks of the consultation in a timely manner.	Consults effectively in a focused manner, moving beyond the essential to take a holistic view of the patient's needs within the time-frame of a normal consultation.
	Aware of when there is a language barrier and can access interpreters either in person or by telephone.	Manages consultations effectively with patients who have different languages, cultures, beliefs and educational backgrounds.	Uses a variety of communication and consultation techniques which demonstrates respect for, and values, diversity.

Data gathering and interpretation

This is about the gathering, interpretation, and use of data for clinical judgement, including information gathered from the history, clinical records, examination and investigations.

Insufficient evidence	Needs further development	Competent	Excellent
From the available evidence, the doctor's performance cannot be placed on a higher point of this developmental scale.	Accumulates information from the patient that is mainly relevant to their problem. Uses existing information in the patient records.	Systematically gathers information, using questions appropriately targeted to the problem without affecting patient safety. Understands the importance of, and makes appropriate use of, existing information about the problem and the patient's context.	Expertly identifies the nature and scope of enquiry needed to investigate the problem, or multiple problems, within a short time-frame. Prioritises problems in a way that enhances patient satisfaction.
	Employs examinations and investigations that are broadly in line with the patient's problems.	Chooses examinations and targets investigations appropriately and efficiently.	Uses a stepwise approach, basing further enquiries, examinations and tests on what is already known and what is later discovered.

3

Insufficient evidence	Needs further development	Competent	Excellent
	Identifies abnormal findings and results.	Understands the significance and implications of findings and results, and takes appropriate action.	
	Demonstrates a limited range of data gathering styles and methods.	Demonstrates different styles of data gathering and adapts these to a wide range of patients and situations.	Able to gather information in a wide range of circumstances and across all patient groups (including their family and representatives) in a sensitive, empathetic and ethical manner.

Making a diagnosis/decisions

This is about a conscious, structured approach to making diagnoses and decision-making.

Insufficient evidence	Needs further development	Competent	Excellent
From the available evidence, the doctor's performance cannot be placed on a higher point of this developmental scale.	Generates an adequate differential diagnosis based on the information available.	Makes diagnoses in a structured way using a problem-solving method. Uses an understanding of probability based on prevalence, incidence and natural history of illness to aid decision-making. Addresses problems that present early and/or in an undifferentiated way by integrating all the available information to help generate a differential diagnosis. Uses time as a diagnostic tool.	Uses pattern recognition to identify diagnoses quickly, safely and reliably. Remains aware of the limitations of pattern recognition and when to revert to an analytical approach.
	Generates and tests appropriate hypotheses.	Revises hypotheses in the light of additional information.	No longer relies on rules or protocols but is able to use and justify discretionary judgement in situations of uncertainty or complexity, for example in patients with multiple problems.
	Makes decisions by applying rules, plans or protocols.	Thinks flexibly around problems generating functional solutions.	

Insufficient evidence	Needs further development	Competent	Excellent
	Asks for help appropriately but fails to progress to making independent decisions.	Has confidence in, and takes ownership of own decisions whilst being aware of their own limitations.	Continues to reflect appropriately on difficult decisions. Develops mechanisms to be comfortable with these choices.
		Keeps an open mind and is able to adjust and revise decisions in the light of relevant new information.	

Clinical management

This is about the recognition and management of patients' problems.

Insufficient evidence	Needs further development	Competent	Excellent
	Uses appropriate but limited management options without taking into account the preferences of the patient.	Varies management options responsively according to the circumstances, priorities and preferences of those involved.	Provides patient-centred management plans whilst taking account of local and national guidelines in a timely manner.
From the available evidence, the doctor's performance cannot be placed on a higher point of this developmental scale.	Suggests intervention in all cases.	Considers a "wait and see" approach where appropriate. Uses effective prioritisation of problems when the patient presents with multiple issues.	Empowers the patient with confidence to manage problems independently together with knowledge of when to seek further help.
	Arranges definite appointments for follow up regardless of need or the nature of the problem.	Suggests a variety of follow-up arrangements that are safe and appropriate, whilst also enhancing patient autonomy.	Able to challenge unrealistic patient expectations and consulting patterns with regard to follow up of current and future problems.

Insufficient evidence	Needs further development	Competent	Excellent
	Makes safe prescribing decisions, routinely checking on drug interactions and side effects.	In addition to prescribing safely, is aware of and applies local and national guidelines including drug and non-drug therapies. Maintains awareness of the legal framework for appropriate prescribing.	Regularly reviews all of the patient's medication in terms of evidence-based prescribing, cost-effectiveness and patient understanding. Has confidence in stopping or stepping down medication where this is appropriate.
	Refers safely, acting within the limits of their competence.	Refers appropriately, taking into account all available resources.	Identifies areas for improvement in referral processes and pathways and contributes to quality improvement.
	Recognises medical emergencies and responds to them safely.	Responds rapidly and skilfully to emergencies, with appropriate follow- up for the patient and their family. Ensures that care is co-ordinated both within the practice team and with other services.	Contributes to reflection on emergencies as significant events and how these can be used to improve patient care in the future.
	Ensures that continuity of care can be provided for the patient's problem, e.g. through adequate record keeping.	Provides comprehensive continuity of care, taking into account all of the patient's problems and their social situation.	Takes active steps within the organisation to improve continuity of care for the patients.

Reproduced from www.rcgp.org.uk/training-exams/mrcgp-workplace-based-assessment-wpba/wpba-competence-framework.aspx with permission.

Why doctors preparing for the CSA should read this book

Preparing for the CSA without an understanding of how to apply the skills recommended in the competency framework, which forms the basis of the grading indicators for the CSA, is a common cause of failure or poor performance. If you look at the table below, the meaning of the competency "uses the patient's understanding to improve the explanation offered" can sometimes be misunderstood by doctors to mean simply the use of 'non-jargon' descriptions of clinical diagnosis. In actual fact, the competency can mean using medical jargon if the use of that language reflects the doctor's understanding of the patient's level of knowledge. For instance, if the doctor believes that the patient understands the medical terminology used, they may well use medical jargon in that consultation to avoid over-simplifying, which may be perceived as patronising by the patient. Using the patient's understanding to help improve the explanation offered is a way for the doctor to show their responsiveness to the understanding of the patient as a person. The CSA assesses the doctor's understanding of the uniqueness of the patient regardless of the nature of the clinical problem presented by the patient. It is clear from the table below that a doctor who is able to provide an explanation that is medically correct and is delivered without the use of medical jargon can still be considered as doctor-centred.

Insufficient evidence	Needs further development	Competent	Excellent
From the available evidence, the doctor's performance cannot be placed on a higher point of this developmental scale.	Provides explanations that are medically correct but doctor-centred.	Uses the patient's understanding to help improve the explanation offered.	Uses a variety of communication techniques and materials (e.g. written or electronic) to adapt explanations to the needs of the patient.

Positive CSA indicators
- Shows responsiveness to the patient's preferences, feelings and expectations.
- Provides explanations that are relevant and understandable to the patient.

If you normally approach data gathering by focusing on the clinical problem presented by the patient, in a bid to make a diagnosis, and then proceed to enquire about the patient's ideas, concerns and expectations, rather than seeking to develop a relationship with the patient, then you need to read this book. The insight in this book will help you to understand the exact meaning of the competencies assessed in the CSA: you are expected to gather data mainly focused on the patient's experience of the problem (to gain an understanding of the uniqueness of the patient's experience), enhancing your ability to focus further enquiries on your understanding of the patient's reasons for attending, and gathering information targeted at both recognising the problem presented by the patient and resolving the patient's main reasons for attending.

Insufficient evidence	Needs further development	Competent	Excellent
	Accumulates information from the patient that is mainly relevant to their problem. Uses existing information in the patient records.	Systematically gathers information, using questions appropriately targeted to the problem without affecting patient safety. Understands the importance of, and makes appropriate use of, existing information about the problem and the patient's context.	Expertly identifies the nature and scope of enquiry needed to investigate the problem, or multiple problems, within a short time-frame. Prioritises problems in a way that enhances patient satisfaction.

It is important that you focus on achieving fluency in patient-centred consulting through repeated practice during real-life encounters. Aim to demonstrate the competencies by practising with real patients in your day-to-day consultations, rather than relying on small group sessions with your peers which are often unable to replicate the uniqueness of the individual patient, which is a key aspect of the competencies assessed in the CSA.

This book helps you to learn how to discover the reasons for the patient's attendance, to understand the patient's perspective, and to use this understanding throughout the consultation. You will learn how to think about the patient rather than focus on the clinical problem and how to show a genuine willingness to explore the patient's world, ultimately achieving the objectives of the consultation more fluently and time-efficiently. This book is structured to mimic a typical consultation, but with a reflection on the thoughts of the doctor to help readers gain more insight into the meaning of the competencies assessed in the CSA.

The three domains of the CSA grading are centred on the doctor's ability to understand and focus on the patient's experience of a problem and their uniqueness rather than just the doctor's understanding of the management of individual disease conditions. This book will help you appreciate how to consult in a way which focuses more on the patient.

Explaining the CSA grading

The CSA examination assesses the ability of the doctor to gather information, apply their understanding of disease processes, make shared decisions and communicate effectively with patients.[1] Because the assessment is divided into three domains, they can be perceived as isolated areas of performance by some candidates, but in fact the domains are interrelated in the skill sets being assessed:

- The data gathering domain requires the doctor to gather information that is targeted to the tasks the patient has presented to resolve (patient's agenda) which is achieved using good interpersonal skills.

- The clinical management domain requires the doctor to tailor their knowledge of the management of common disease presentations to reflect their understanding of the uniqueness of the patient's experience and their context; this also requires good interpersonal skills.

If the doctor approaches the consultation mainly focused on gathering data related to the clinical condition, they may not achieve this level of focus, even if they eventually enquire as to the patient's ideas, concerns and expectations at some stage in the consultation. The consultation may not then have been focused and logical, follow the patient from their train, or their reasons for attending, to build a therapeutic and empathetic relationship with them. This ability to show responsiveness to the patient's views and preferences by tailoring the approach so that the doctor can offer the patient appropriate and feasible options is reflected in all the three domains of the CSA assessment.

Clinical management skills positive indicators
- Offers appropriate and feasible management options.
- Is cooperative and inclusive in approach.
- Shows responsiveness to the patient's preferences, feelings and expectations.
- Works in partnership, finding common ground to develop a shared management plan.

Common reasons for failure in the CSA

Doctors fail the CSA because they have not developed fluency in patient-centredness.[2] This fluency is achieved by practising the skills in real life using the right understanding of the competencies as they should be applied. Commonly, the doctor has not focused their exam preparation on the understanding of the patient, but mainly on the clinical problem presented, and therefore does not achieve the level of fluency required to perform at a competent level. The reasons for failure in the CSA as published by the RCGP[1] highlight these problems, as outlined below.

This book addresses each of these common problems using typical consultation dialogues to demonstrate how to use these skills in the consultation to build a relationship with the patient.

Wrong approach to the consultation – failure to focus on the patient

Doctor: *"What brings you here today?"*

Patient: *"It's this lump on my wrist, doctor."*

Every patient will have a specific reason for attending with their symptom or problem. They may have tried to work out what the problem is, or considered how best they feel it should be dealt with. Patients have an idea about how the problem is affecting them, and what concerns them about it. These aspects of the patient's experience can be discovered more effectively by encouraging them to share their views without any interruptions. These interruptions can be in any form, such as the doctor choosing lines of enquiry which distract the patient from their line of thought by focusing mainly on the problem, or not being open enough to allow the patient to share their views. This information is important in achieving patient-centredness, because the doctor is able to understand far better the nature of the condition the patient has presented with, by listening carefully to the individual patient's experience. The doctor is less likely to make any assumptions about the problem, but will be able to clarify the reasons why the patient has attended and help resolve any decisions jointly with them.

Negative CSA indicator
- Makes immediate assumptions about the problem.

Doctor: *"Can you tell me what's happened?"*

Open question aimed at exploring the patient's own experience. The doctor should concentrate at this stage on understanding the patient's experience of the problem, to build a relationship based on shared understanding, whilst also recognising the pattern of the common condition presented within that context. The ability to recognise the clinical problem in this way is the basis of the fluency and focus recommended by the RCGP, and achieving this fluency helps prevent the doctor from being illogical and disjointed in their consultation.

> **Positive CSA indicators**
> - Recognises presentations of common physical, psychological and social problems.
> - Data gathering appears to be guided by the probabilities of disease.

Patient: *"I noticed it about a week ago. It just came on for no apparent reason, and has remained the same size since then. I'm really not sure what it could be."*

The patient's account gives the doctor an indication of what they may have been thinking about the problem, and also presents an opportunity for the doctor to explore the patient's own understanding by observing verbal cues. Acquiring this information helps the doctor to focus the consultation on addressing the issues the patient has attended with. It's difficult to achieve a partnership without sufficiently exploring and understanding the patient's own views and thoughts about the situation.

Doctor: *"How does the area feel?"*

Focused on the problem and this distracts the patient from their train of thought. In some cases, a clarification such as this may be necessary initially for the doctor to recognise the problem, but in this case asking the reason for the patient's attendance is more important to allow the doctor to focus their data gathering on the patient.

Insufficient evidence	Needs further development	Competent	Excellent
	Accumulates information from the patient that is mainly relevant to their problem. Uses existing information in the patient records.	Systematically gathers information, using questions appropriately targeted to the problem without affecting patient safety. Understands the importance of, and makes appropriate use of, existing information about the problem and the patient's context.	Expertly identifies the nature and scope of enquiry needed to investigate the problem, or multiple problems, within a short time-frame. Prioritises problems in a way that enhances patient satisfaction.

> **Positive CSA indicators**
> - Clarifies the problem and nature of the decision required.
> - Uses an incremental approach, using time and accepting uncertainty.
>
> **Negative CSA indicators**
> - Makes immediate assumptions about the problem.
> - Is disorganised/unsystematic in gathering information.

Patient: *"It's not painful at all, and hasn't given me any problems really. It just doesn't look good where it is."*

The patient is responding directly to the doctor's question rather than sharing their own thoughts. This line of questioning may distract the patient from their own train of thought or the issue they attended to focus on (preference).

Doctor: *"What do you think has caused it?"*

Doctor seeks to clarify the patient's ideas. It is usually more effective to allow the patient to share their thoughts: they may, for instance, have some ideas but have not considered or seen these ideas as causes. They are more likely to share those thoughts in the context of an open exploration of their views by using reflective questioning to guide them.

> *Negative CSA indicator*
> - Pays insufficient attention to the patient's verbal and non-verbal communication.

Patient: *"I'm not really sure."*

The doctor has not shown a willingness to encourage the patient's contribution, and has used a formulaic ICE question that is often not as useful as a reflective question which is in the context of the patient's thoughts. Patients respond better when the approach is aimed at building a relationship and rapport, focusing on the patient's own experience and views.

Doctor: *"Has it affected your job?"*

Again, the doctor does not follow the line of thought of the patient to develop an insight into the reason for the patient's attendance, or to try to appreciate the impact of the problem through that context. Questions asked out of context without demonstrating an understanding of the patient's story are not likely to enhance the relationship or rapport building. The patient's opening statement suggested that they were puzzled about this lump and so they may have thought about the nature of it. Following that line of thought using reflective questioning is more likely to open up the 'life world' of the patient's experience and improve the shared understanding of the direction of the consultation.

Patient: *"Not really."*

The patient is responding to a question which does not provide them with an opportunity to share their experience and views.

Doctor: *"What were you hoping I would be able to do about it for you?"*

Doctor seeking to explore the patient's expectations using a formulaic question. Some patients may share their expectations from the consultation at this stage, but others often feel that they are being asked to dictate the outcome of the consultation. Patients feel more able to share their thoughts when the approach is inclusive and open, and their views and thoughts have been invited using reflective questions which demonstrate active listening.

> *Negative CSA indicator*
> - Uses a rigid approach to consulting that fails to be sufficiently responsive to the patient's contribution.

Patient: *"I'd like to get rid of it if possible."*

The patient is simply responding to the doctor's direct question rather than becoming a partner in the consultation. They should have been encouraged to share their views and within that context the doctor would gain more insight into the patient's expectations and preferences, whilst at the same time recognising the clinical condition presented. The question the doctor asked looks to have been too narrow to give the patient an opportunity to express their thoughts, preferences and views. The doctor is not being guided by the patient's own account of the problem and so does not develop a relationship with the patient (rapport building).

Negative CSA indicators
- Does not inquire sufficiently about the patient's perspective/health understanding.
- Pays insufficient attention to the patient's verbal and non-verbal communication.

Doctor: *"Does anything particularly worry you about it?"*

Formulaic question to explore patient's concerns. Although most patients have something that particularly concerns them about a problem, they may not necessarily understand the intention of the question when it is asked in this way. Some patients may misunderstand the question as being an enquiry into the severity of the problem or perhaps, as in this case, they may feel they shouldn't really be concerned about a trivial problem like a ganglion. Some patients may have thoughts about a problem but may not have perceived those thoughts as worries, as put in the question. Rather, the doctor should have developed this understanding through encouraging the patient to share their thoughts and views.

Negative CSA indicator
- Does not appreciate the impact of the patient's psychosocial context.

Patient: *"Not really."*

Ineffective enquiry. The patient may have been able to share their experiences more if they were given an opportunity to share their own thoughts and feelings.

Doctor: *"OK, before we discuss how to manage it, I would like to ask you some specific questions to help me understand your general health. Is that OK?"*

Negative CSA indicator
- Makes immediate assumptions about the task.

Doctor: *"Do you have any other health problems? Does anyone else in your family have anything similar? Do you smoke? Do you take any medicines?"*

Closed questions appropriately used, but the questions should be guided by the understanding of the probability of the likely disease and should be logical. It should reflect the doctor's ability to recognise a common condition and show their understanding of the natural course of the condition.

Negative CSA indicator
- Data gathering does not appear to be guided by the main task the patient presented to resolve.

Doctor: *"Is it OK if I have a look at the wrist?"*

Examination: ganglion; normal wrist movement.

Doctor: *"From the examination, the lump looks like what we call a ganglion. These are small cysts that can come off a tendon, often for no specific reason. They're not normally harmful and don't usually cause any pain or problems."*

The explanation is medically correct and given without using jargon, but fails to take into account the patient's reason for attending (you will see this in the 'right approach' section below). The CSA is designed to assess the doctor's ability to explore and respond to the uniqueness of the problem to the patient, working in partnership with them to find a common ground by using their learned knowledge and interpretation of the problem in the context of the patient. The explanation should reflect the doctor's understanding of the patient.

Negative CSA indicators
- Uses a rigid approach to consulting that fails to be sufficiently responsive to the patient's contribution.
- Provides explanations that do not reflect an understanding of the patient.

Doctor: *"It would usually be better not to do anything, because often they resolve on their own. If they begin to cause you problems or any pain, then perhaps we can refer you to a surgeon to consider removing them, but you need to be aware that they can recur after they've been removed. Are you OK with that?"*

The doctor is giving options but without taking into account the patient's thoughts and experience. Although the doctor seeks to get the agreement of the patient here, it is less effective than if the patient's views were taken into account during the decision-making.

Negative CSA indicators
- Instructs the patient rather than seeking common ground.
- Uses a rigid approach to consulting that fails to be sufficiently responsive to the patient's contribution.

Patient: *"With my wrist like this, do you think it's OK to continue playing tennis, or would that be a problem?"*

Verbal cue late, poor rapport, patient not involved in the decision-making.

Doctor: *"How often do you play tennis?"*

Disjointed consultation and with poor time management.

Negative CSA indicators
- Makes immediate assumptions about the problem.
- Intervenes rather than using appropriate expectant management.
- Is disorganised/unsystematic in gathering information.
- Data gathering does not appear to be guided by the probabilities of disease.

Patient: *"I play professionally and I represent the whole of the south-east. I've been training really hard for the last few months, but can't remember hurting myself at all."*

Patient's perspective and experience of the problem realised late.

Doctor: *"Does it give you any problems when you play?"*

Disjointed again. Discovered main issue late because the doctor did not clarify the reason for the patient's attendance at the outset.

> **Negative CSA indicator**
> * Is disorganised/unsystematic in gathering information.

Patient: *"I haven't really played tennis since I noticed it, because I thought I'd get you to check it out first before I restarted playing."*

Patient's experience offered late.

Doctor: *"I don't think there is any reason why you shouldn't be able to play, but if it bothers you while playing, you can let me have a look at it again."*

Poor rapport. Difficult to empathise appropriately.

Patient: *"I know you said they can disappear on their own without any treatment, but is there anything I can do to help the process go a little quicker?"*

Patient's concerns and expectations, verbal cues late.

Doctor: *"Is there a particular reason you would like it to get better quicker?"*

Disjointed and failing to take account of patient's previous answers.

Patient: *"The south-east tennis team is very competitive, and I've done a lot of training to get to the level I am now. I wouldn't want anything like this to jeopardise my progress, and once my coach sees my wrist, it's possible they may not select me for the final which is coming up soon. They may need a written note to say my wrist is OK, and that it won't affect my game."*

Reason for attending.

> **Negative CSA indicators**
> * Does not inquire sufficiently about the patient's perspective/health understanding.
> * Fails to explore how the patient's life is affected by the problem.
> * Does not appreciate the impact of the patient's psychosocial context.
> * Does not work in partnership.

Doctor: *"OK."*

The doctor fails to clarify the main issue the patient needs help with because they did not focus on developing a relationship with the patient based on encouraging them to share their thoughts and experience of the problem. The consultation was not guided by clarification of the main reason for the patient's attendance or the nature of the decision the patient wanted to address. The doctor does not enhance the patient's autonomy to participate in the decision related to their own health concerns, and the doctor does not show responsiveness to the patient's experience, feelings and preferences.

> **Positive CSA indicators**
> * Responds to needs and concerns with interest and understanding.
> * Shows responsiveness to the patient's preferences, feelings and expectations.
> * Enhances patient autonomy.

Right approach to the consultation – focusing on the patient

This book explores how to solve the common causes of failure in the CSA. The dialogue below applies the CSA competencies required by the RCGP, to show how the doctor can work in partnership with the patient to achieve a successful consultation by understanding the patient's perspective of the problem, and not focusing mainly on the problem.

Doctor: *"What brings you here today?"*

Patient: *"It's this lump on my wrist, doctor."*

Doctor: *"Can you tell me what has happened?"*

Patient: *"I noticed it about a week ago. It just came on for no apparent reason, and has remained the same size since then. I'm not really sure what it could be exactly."*

Doctor: *"It must have been a little surprising for you that it's just appeared."*

Reflective questioning here helps to encourage the patient's contribution to understanding their unique experience of the problem, clarify their reasons for attending and the nature of the decision to be made. The doctor is seeking to allow the patient to explore their inner thoughts and to gain more insight into their 'life world'. This context is an important part of the CSA assessment, because understanding it allows the doctor to empathise more appropriately, to be able to tailor the information they offer, the management options they discuss, their data gathering around the problem, and to build good rapport with the patient using their understanding of the patient's unique experience.

> *Positive CSA indicators*
> - Explores patient's agenda, health beliefs and preferences.
> - Appears alert to verbal and non-verbal cues.
> - Explores the impact of the illness on the patient's life.
> - Elicits psychological and social information to place the patient's problem in context.
> - Is cooperative and inclusive in approach.

Patient: *"It was, because I just couldn't pinpoint if there were things I was doing differently to bring it on. It just came up one morning and I thought perhaps it would go down but it has remained exactly the same. It's not painful or anything but doesn't look like it's shifting."*

Verbal cues. Patient expresses their line of thoughts regarding the problem because they feel empowered to share their inner feelings about the problem in the consultation. This aspect of the consultation is a common reason for CSA failure if the doctor does not learn how to explore the patient's perspective, as you will see in the rest of the book.

Doctor: *"I can see that this bothers you a bit."*

Responding to verbal cues aimed at developing the patient's understanding. Active listening (the doctor understood from the patient's description that they sounded a little bit frustrated that the lump had remained). Building the history of the problem from the perspective of the patient's experience of it. Encouraging the patient's contribution, by showing willingness to listen to their thoughts and feelings in a non-formulaic manner.

Insufficient evidence	Needs further development	Competent	Excellent
	Develops a relationship with the patient, which works, but is focused on the problem rather than the patient.	Explores and responds to the patient's agenda, health beliefs and preferences. Elicits psychological and social information to place the patient's problem in context.	Incorporates the patient's perspective and context when negotiating the management plan.

Patient: *"Normally things like this don't bother me, but I'm a tennis player and have been preparing for a tournament. I was a tiny bit bothered when I noticed the lump come up, but I'm hoping that it isn't anything that should really affect my game."*

Positive CSA indicator
- Elicits psychological and social information to place the patient's problem in context.

Doctor: *"It sounds like you were worried about the effect it might have on your performance."*

Doctor responding to verbal cues to gain more insight into the patient's concerns and the impact of the problem on the patient. This information is likely to place the problem in the right context of the patient's world, providing the basis for a mutual agreement.

Patient: *"Although one of my friends said this could be a ganglion, I still feel the coach may decide to drop me from the team as pressure for places is getting a bit intense now. I thought perhaps if I can get it confirmed as a ganglion then either I can get it removed or get a note to show to the coach that it isn't something that will affect my game."*

Patient now appears to be contributing their views more readily because of the rapport developed by the open approach of the doctor and their willingness to encourage the patient to share those views using active listening and reflective questioning.

Positive CSA indicators
- Clarifies the problem and nature of decision required.
- Uses an incremental approach, using time and accepting uncertainty.
- Gathers information from history taking, examination and investigation in a systematic and efficient manner.

Doctor: *"I can understand why that would worry you. I'm going to ask you some specific questions to understand the lump a bit better – is that OK?"*

Empathy.

Positive CSA indicators
- Explores the impact of the illness on the patient's life.
- Elicits psychological and social information to place the patient's problem in context.

The doctor uses closed questions to clarify a possible history of trauma from playing tennis, to clarify effects during play, verifies the timing of the tournament, checks drug history.

Focused history taking demonstrates an understanding of the main task. The doctor is selective with their questions, using an understanding of likelihood and probabilities, and follows a logical line of enquiry showing their understanding of the task the patient has presented to resolve. The doctor also uses closed questions, guided by their knowledge of probabilities based on prevalence and likelihood and accepting uncertainties, to make a diagnosis, rather than exhaustive questioning without showing acceptance of uncertainty.

Positive CSA indicators
- Uses an incremental approach, using time and accepting uncertainty.
- Is appropriately selective in the choice of enquiries, examinations and investigations.

Doctor: *"Is it OK if I have a look at your wrist?"*

Examination: Ganglion. Normal wrist movement.

Doctor: *"I can confirm that you're right – it is a ganglion. They are cysts that can come up on their own around the wrist. It sounds like the cyst has become more prominent since you started the intensive training, but you haven't hurt yourself particularly so we can't really say for sure if this has anything to do with the training. Your wrist movement is normal so I wouldn't expect you to have any problems playing tennis, unless you start noticing soreness or pain around the area."*

Using the understanding of the patient's experience to improve the explanation offered. The doctor responds to their understanding of the problem and the patient. This ability to respond to the explored perspective of the patient is at the heart of the CSA grading, because it shows the doctor's responsiveness to the patient's preference and thoughts.

Insufficient evidence	Needs further development	Competent	Excellent
	Develops a relationship with the patient, which works, but is focused on the problem rather than the patient.	Explores and responds to the patient's agenda, health beliefs and preferences. Elicits psychological and social information to place the patient's problem in context.	Incorporates the patient's perspective and context when negotiating the management plan.

Positive CSA indicators
- Enhances patient autonomy.
- Provides explanations that are relevant and understandable to the patient.
- Shows responsiveness to the patient's preferences, feelings and expectations.

Doctor: *"I know you were wondering about removing the cyst. This would normally require a referral to the hospital, and it would take a few months to get an appointment to see one of the surgeons if you wanted to take this route. Sometimes they can resolve on their own without having to have any surgery, but this can take up to a year or so. I know the tournament is really important to you right now, but I'm not sure if there's anything that can be done in this short period before that."*

Offering advice using the doctor's understanding of the patient and their preferences. Taking into account the patient's concerns and their reason for attending. The doctor recognised the nature of the decision the patient has attended to make.

Positive CSA indicators
- Works in partnership, finding common ground to develop a shared management plan.
- Communicates risk effectively to patients.
- Shows responsiveness to the patient's preferences, feelings and expectations.

Positive indicators of management skills
- Recognises presentations of common physical, psychological and social problems.
- Makes plans that reflect the natural history of common problems.
- Offers appropriate and feasible management options.

Patient: *"Perhaps I could just have to hand a written note to give to the coach if you don't think it will affect my play."*

Doctor: *"I'm happy to support you with that as I don't see any reason you can't continue with your training, but it would be a good idea to let me know if you start experiencing any problems or pain while playing."*

Achieving the task of the consultation by responding to the reason for the patient's attendance. This reduces the occurrence of discordance as observed in the first dialogue. The rapport is better and the doctor empathises more appropriately using their understanding of the patient. The patient feels more empowered because their views and thoughts have been taken into account in the decision-making process.

Positive CSA indicators
- Responds to needs and concerns with interest and understanding.
- Works in partnership with the patient negotiating a mutual plan.
- Uses an incremental approach, using time and accepting uncertainties.

Insufficient evidence	Needs further development	Competent	Excellent
	Communicates management plans but without negotiating with, or involving, the patient.	Works in partnership with the patient, negotiating a mutually acceptable plan that respects the patient's agenda and preference for involvement.	Whenever possible, adopts plans that respect the patient's autonomy. When there is a difference of opinion the patient's autonomy is respected and a positive relationship is maintained.

The doctor explores the patient's perspective by encouraging the patient's contribution using active listening and reflective questions to gain an insight into the patient's unique experience of the problem. Within that context, the doctor understands the patient's thoughts, experience, preferences, reason for attending, and the nature of the decision they have attended to make. The doctor responds to this understanding, from the explanation they offered, the way they tailored the options of treatment offered, and the nature of specific safety netting agreed. The doctor achieved the task of the consultation working in partnership with the patient to find a mutually agreed plan.

Exploring the reasons for failure

Disorganised/unstructured consultation

If the doctor does not discover the nature of the patient's experience of a problem and so understand the reasons why the patient has attended, they may spend a lot of time focusing on the clinical problem presented by the patient rather than getting information that is relevant to the patient, which allows the doctor to assist the patient in making the appropriate decisions. The doctor may then continue to gather data in the management stages because the patient's agenda only becomes apparent late in the consultation – this is time-inefficient and makes the consultation appear disjointed. The doctor should use selective questions that are logical and show an understanding of the problems presented by the patient, rather than using broad exhaustive questions which may be out of context. The data gathering should be guided by the patient's experience of the problem and also the doctor's knowledge of the likely cause of their problem based on probability. The line of enquiry should be one that is logical and follows the line of thought of the patient and their agenda. It is clear that underlying this failure is the inadequate exploration of the patient's experience and perspective. The consultation cannot be patient-centred if the doctor does not develop an understanding of the patient as a whole and just focuses on the clinical problem – this leaves the doctor unable to be selective and systematic in their approach. This problem is solved by the doctor learning how to show willingness to encourage the patient's contribution during the encounter using an inclusive and open approach.

Does not recognise the issues or priorities

The main reason why the patient has attended was missed in the "wrong approach" consultation because the doctor was unable to sufficiently explore the patient's agenda and preferences. They were not able to encourage the patient to share those thoughts within the data gathering stages, and therefore unable to achieve the main tasks in partnership with the patient. This does not mean that the patient had a hidden agenda, but the style of the doctor wasn't open and inclusive enough to encourage the patient's contribution early in the consultation. The doctor did not develop a relationship with the patient which was based on their understanding of the patient's perspective. For example, a patient who presented with a ganglion and wanted to discuss if he could get a note to reassure his coach that he would be OK to play in an upcoming important tournament, may have required a focus on examination of their wrist with a view to advising them on the tournament, but in this case the doctor assumed the patient had attended to get a diagnosis and treatment of their ganglion. They did not recognise the patient's agenda issues because they did not sufficiently explore the patient perspective or encourage the patient's contribution in the consultation.

Shows poor time management

The doctor had not practised patient-centredness enough in training to become fluent and efficient. They have not become selective enough in their line of enquiry, in response to a recognition of the nature of the clinical problem presented, and the reasons for the patient's attendance or the nature of the decision required. This lack of focus causes the doctor to spend time on areas of the consultation that may not necessarily be of any use to either the patient or the management of the clinical problem presented. This focus is mostly learned from regular practice using the right understanding of the competencies rather than just case-based rehearsal before the examination.

Does not appear to develop rapport or show awareness of the patient's agenda and preferences

This happens when the doctor approaches the consultation without an understanding of how to work in partnership with the patient. They do not understand how to gather information from the patient's perspective, guiding the patient to share their thoughts and views about their problem without using narrow interview-type questions which are not exploratory enough. They are not able to recognise the reason the patient has attended through a systematic exploration of the patient's experience of the problem. They use formulaic questions to gather information related to the patient's experience which are often out of context and may not build a relationship which is based on a shared understanding of each other's feelings. The doctor focuses on the clinical 'problem', rather than the patient's experience of the problem, during their preparation for the examination. This book explores all aspects of the patient's perspective, demonstrating how the doctor can build rapport by working in partnership with the patient throughout the consultation.

Poor active listening skills and use of cues

This happens when the doctor does not use a line of enquiry which demonstrates to the patient that they understood what they have said, using reflective statements and questions to encourage the patient to share their own views. The doctor's questioning indicates a poor understanding of the patient's line of thought and this often happens when the doctor focuses mainly on the clinical problem rather than on developing an understanding of the patient's experience of the problem.

Does not develop a shared plan

In the "wrong approach" consultation above, the doctor did not enquire sufficiently into the patient's own experience of the problem to enable them to develop an understanding of the patient's views and beliefs. This means that they cannot find a basis for a mutual negotiation and shared decision-making. The doctor's approach is not inclusive enough to invite the patient to express their feelings about their problem and their thoughts about the treatment options offered. They are not suggestive enough in the options of management they offer, and their choice of treatment options does not reflect their understanding of the patient's perspective and preferences. This lack of responsiveness to the patient's feelings and preferences is considered as "doctor-centredness" in the CSA examination.

Does not use language that is relevant and understandable to the patient

The doctor is unable to explain the problem using their understanding of the patient's perspective. Some doctors rehearse how to explain medical conditions using jargon-free language, rather than focusing on offering explanations which reflect their understanding of the nature of the information the patient needs and the uniqueness of the individual. They have not shown responsiveness to the patient's ideas and preferences and have not empowered the patient by improving the patient's understanding of the problem.

It should be clear from the reasons outlined above (and the exam feedback published by the RCGP) that the common causes of CSA failure are not usually due to the doctor's lack of clinical knowledge. Instead, failures are often due to poor fluency in applying that knowledge and in responding and showing an awareness of the uniqueness of the individual patient and their experience of the problem. In other words, the doctor is not patient-centred in their approach, and this is usually as a result of misunderstanding the competencies assessed in the CSA.

Recommended approach to help you pass the CSA

This book explores several aspects of the RCGP competency framework, to enhance the achievement of patient-centredness by guiding the doctor through the inner thoughts of a clinician working at the level expected in the CSA using real-life patient–doctor dialogues. Doctors are expected to adopt a style of consultation from one of the established patient-centred models of consultation, i.e. Helman, Pendleton or Neighbour[3], practising to become fluent in their use. In the CSA, the doctor is expected to consult in a way that reflects an approach which they have mastered and adopted to suit their individual styles. This book is based on an approach which directly addresses what the CSA is designed to assess, using a structure which can be applied flexibly to any case regardless of the clinical problem presented.

In this book, I have explored an approach which achieves patient-centredness by focusing the consultation around the uniqueness of the patient, especially if that understanding of the patient's perspective is achieved in the early stages of the consultation.

This approach will assist the doctor in learning how to build a therapeutic rapport with the patient, efficiently clarify the reason for the patient's attendance, and establish a therapeutic empathetic relationship with the patient. It will also demonstrate how to achieve a coherent consultation, a true partnership with the patient (in a **timely and efficient** manner to empower the patient), and a safe shared management plan.[2]

Recommended structure to achieve patient-centredness in the CSA

Stage A
- Allow the patient to tell their story, or facilitate the process using active listening to understand and recognise the clinical problem through the experience of the patient.
- Explore the patient's understanding, feelings and preferences using reflective questions and active listening to put the problem in context, understanding its impact on the patient within that context.
- Establish rapport using active listening and empathy, gathering information which shows you are preparing to find a common ground for negotiation.
- Clarify the reason for attending, discover the main tasks, recognise the clinical problem and the nature of the decision to be made through its description by the patient.

Aim to achieve fluency in your day-to-day consultations. Use flexibility to decide which enquiry comes first, responding to the style of the patient and nature of the problem. Summarise or paraphrase to check understanding.

Stage B
- Use closed questions to focus the history to the problem, using a knowledge of probability based on prevalence to clarify the diagnosis, accepting uncertainties and using time as a tool in an incremental manner.
- Exclude red flags to address both patient and doctor agendas.
- Focused examination which is selective enough to address doctor and patient concerns.

Use signposting to move from one section to another.

Stage C
- Explain the problem to show responsiveness to the patient's preference, feelings and expectations.

Don't simply use generic non-medical jargon, tailor the explanation to the patient using your understanding of their reason for attending.

Stage D
- Discuss possible options, responding to the understanding of the patient's perspective in an incremental order. Safety netting to reflect an understanding of the risks/uncertainties of consulting in a focused way.

Think feasible and relevant, not just all the management steps.

This approach helps the doctor to achieve patient-centredness efficiently, and to develop a logical and coherent consultation as required when demonstrating a satisfactory skill level in the CSA examination. The structure provides a working guide for the doctor to build on their understanding of the competencies as explored in detail in this book.

An example of the use of the recommended approach and how the positive indicators are scored

Stage A

Patient: *"I just feel so down, doctor."*

Doctor: *"Please tell me what's been happening."*

Open question.

Patient: *"I just can't find the motivation to do anything, everything seems to be an effort for me to do now. Even getting up in the morning is getting very difficult as it feels like there is really no point. It just feels like there is a cloud over my head, and I've been trying to use all the skills I learnt from CBT to help the situation, but it just seems like nothing is changing no matter what I do. I really do think perhaps this is the right time to talk to someone about it."*

Recognising a common condition from the pattern and description. Active listening to understand the patient's thoughts and experience, observing verbal cues.

- Recognises presentations of common physical, psychological and social problems.

Doctor: *"I think you've done well to attend to talk about it. Can you tell me what's been going on in your head?"*

Positive attitude, open and inclusive in approach. Reflective questioning based on active listening to encourage the patient to share their thoughts.

- Clarifies the problem and nature of decision required.

- Has a positive attitude when dealing with problems, admits mistakes and shows commitment to improvement.

Patient: *"I've been planning to emigrate to France for the last year, and although it's something that I would like to do, it seems more difficult to think about it as the time to do it is getting closer and closer. It's not that I'm afraid of making the trip but it just feels a little overwhelming sometimes to think about it."*

Patient able to share their thoughts without having to answer direct questions at this stage. The doctor is able to understand the main reason for attending.

Doctor: *"It definitely sounds like a very important decision for you. Why France and when are you planning to move?"*

Selective question based on the doctor's understanding of the probable cause of the problem. Clarifying the reason for attending and understanding the context.

- Explores the patient's agenda, health beliefs and preferences.

Patient: *"I'm hoping to move over in the next 4 weeks as all my friends live in France and have done for a few years now. I don't have any friends in the UK. I know that they will give me accommodation for at least 2 months once I arrive, and I intend to get a job to take care of myself when I'm there. The prospect of getting there and things perhaps not working out well is an overwhelming thought."*

The doctor understands the context of their problem but the decision they need help to resolve remains unclear.

Doctor: *"It sounds like this has been a difficult decision for you to make. You said that you have had CBT previously. Have you suffered from previous problems with your mental health?"*

Empathy. Understands the impact of the situation on the patient, exploring verbal cues to gain understanding of the patient's experience and put the current complaint in the context of that experience. Holistic view.

- Explores the patient's agenda, health beliefs and preferences.

- Appears alert to verbal and non-verbal cues.

Patient: *"I was seeing a therapist 2 years ago, when I lost my mother. I had several sessions of therapy which were very helpful at the time, but I was also put on mirtazapine which I take once every night and still do today. The medication effect I think has plateaued out, but it is definitely still helping because when I have stopped it a few times in the past, I got even more anxious."*

Patient's understanding and health beliefs. Establishing a patient's understanding of potential treatment options prepares the doctor to find a common ground during negotiation. This is achieved by pre-empting the nature of discussion to come using an early recognition of the problem presented and verbal cues.

Doctor: *"Were you considering having any support from counselling to help you through the difficulties that you are experiencing now?"*

Verbal cues from previous comment. Clarifying the reason for attending and the nature of the decision to be made.

- Explores the patient's agenda, health beliefs and preferences.

- Appears alert to verbal and non-verbal cues.

- Clarifies the problem and nature of decision required.

Patient: *"I'd like to have a chance to discuss the way I'm feeling with a counsellor, just to put my mind at rest that it's normal to feel this way. I'm not feeling as bad as I was a couple of years ago, but I would like to discuss perhaps changing the antidepressant that I'm taking now to a different type to see if it would help my feelings more. I also wondered if it was possible to speak to someone who can advise me on the risks of the move with regards to my benefits in the UK."*

Patient's expectation realised without using formulaic question, but by efficiently exploring the patient's experience through encouraging them to share their views using active listening and reflective questions.

Doctor: *"Did you have any particular medication in mind, or were you just thinking that a change might help?"*

Patient: *"Two of my friends are on citalopram and they feel that they've benefited from it a lot."*

Patient's ideas. Doctor uses this shared understanding to work in partnership with the patient during shared decision-making.

Doctor: *"What is your current living situation in the UK?"*

Opportunistic and question asked in context. Establishing context and social information.

- Is appropriately selective in the choice of enquiries, examinations and investigations.

Patient: *"I work 16 hours a week, and receive support from the DWP in the form of tax credit. I'm not married and currently live with my father who is a pensioner. I manage quite well with my finances here, but have always wanted to learn French. I intend to use my English language as a skill in France when I move, but would need to learn the French language first before I would be able to get any job there. This is what most of my friends do in France now."*

The doctor puts the problem into context, and develops an understanding of the person, not just the disease. It is clear that the doctor has focused their enquiry on developing a relationship with the patient to gain a shared understanding of their reasons for attending, and is able to focus the rest of the consultation on achieving this task in a systematic and non-disjointed way.

- Elicits psychological and social information to place the patient's problem in context.

Doctor: *"I know that you said things are not as bad as they were 2 years ago, but can you tell me how you have been coping with your day-to-day activities?"*

Severity and risk assessment.

- Explores the impact of the illness on the patient's life.

Patient: *"I still manage to go into work, and there hasn't been any problem on that front. I enjoy playing chess and still go to the local club every Tuesday. There haven't been any problems with my sleeping or with eating, unlike 2 years ago, when it became so bad that I lost my appetite and really struggled to sleep."*

Doctor: *"I know things have been quite difficult for you over this time, but can you tell me the lowest point it has got to since then?"*

Reflective questioning. Risk assessment and making a diagnosis.

- Gathers information from history taking, examination and investigation in a systematic and efficient manner.

- Is appropriately selective in the choice of enquiries, examinations and investigations.

Patient: *"I have had some days when I've felt really very low, to a point that it just feels like the world has come to a standstill, but I haven't had any thoughts of suicide or anything like that. I'm not the sort of person to do that sort of thing. I am an only child, and I wouldn't contemplate doing such a thing to my father."*

Stage B

Doctor uses closed questions to clarify his general health, reviews his drug history, and relevant PMH. Allergies. Alcohol and smoking history.

Doctor: *"Is it OK if I ask you some questions just to give me an idea of your mental state?"*

Examination: PHQ-9 = 7. Mirtazapine 45 mg.

Diagnosis: *Stress and anxiety on a background of depression.*

Stage C

Doctor: *"I know things have been difficult for you, and I can see how the prospect of what sounds like a major life change is affecting you. I think you've done the right thing to seek help and support in making a decision in this situation."*

Explaining the problem using their understanding of the patient's experience. It is important to note that the doctor has recognised this consultation was not about making a diagnosis of depression or to explain a diagnosis of depression to the patient in lay terms. The doctor recognised the exact reason why the patient has attended and has made a clinical diagnosis of an effect on his previous health by the recent life change. The doctor has then explained this to the patient using information which shows their understanding of the patient's experience of the problem and the reason for their attendance.

- Recognises presentations of common physical, psychological and social problems.

- Shows responsiveness to the patient's preferences, feelings and expectations.

- Enhances patient autonomy.

- Provides explanations that are relevant and understandable to the patient.

Stage D

Doctor: *"With regard to your medication, you're currently on the highest dose of mirtazapine. I know you had considered trying a different type of antidepressant, which I think is a reasonable thought, but I'm not sure if you're aware that they are all similar in their effectiveness – although different types can be more helpful to certain people. Citalopram is certainly a very effective treatment for depression, but it's important to remember that these medications can take 3–4 weeks to have any effect and I know your trip is just 4 weeks away. I'm not sure whether you've considered the prospects of making such a change now and whether you feel it would be a good time, especially if you have been fine on the medication for many years. It seems that the move to France has been the major trigger for the way you feel now."*

Explaining the options using the doctor's understanding of the patient's perspectives. Giving options in incremental steps but tailored to the patient's unique situation and not just a generic description of how to manage depression.

- Uses an incremental approach, using time and accepting uncertainty.

- Makes plans that reflect the natural history of common problems.

- Offers appropriate and feasible management options.

- Simultaneously manages multiple health problems, both acute and chronic.

- Provides explanations that are relevant and understandable to the patient.

Patient: *"I can understand what you mean, and I had forgotten that the medication can take that long to have an effect. You're right about the effect the trip is having on my mind. Do you think perhaps it would be better to speak to someone first?"*

- Works in partnership, finding common ground to develop a shared management plan.

Doctor: *"I think it might be helpful to share your feelings and thoughts about the prospect of moving to France with a counsellor. This should help you understand your emotions better and possibly gain an insight that will put you in a stronger position to cope better with the decision you make."*

Shared decision and partnership. The doctor does not simply offer an option of counselling but shares their thoughts using their understanding of the patient's thoughts.

- Makes plans that reflect the natural history of common problems.

- Offers appropriate and feasible management options.

Patient: *"It sounds like a good idea to do that first."*

Mutual understanding due to a sharing of thoughts and negotiation.

Doctor: *"With regards to your benefits, I wondered whether it would be a good idea to speak to the Citizens Advice Bureau to get some advice on how the change in circumstances would affect your benefits going forwards."*

Signposting.

Patient: *"OK, that sounds like a good idea."*

Doctor: *"I can arrange for you to see a counsellor within the next few weeks to go through these thoughts and feelings you are experiencing. In the meantime, we've agreed to continue on your mirtazapine, so that we don't rock the boat while things are changing for you. It would be a good idea for you to come back in to see me before you travel to discuss how you got on with the counsellor and CAB, and so that we can see if there is anything further that we can do to support you. In the meantime, if you ever feel overwhelmed or feel that you are struggling more, you must let me know."*

- Manages risk effectively, safety netting appropriately.

- Uses an incremental approach, using time and accepting uncertainty.

- Makes plans that reflect the natural history of common problems.

- Responds to needs and concerns with interest and understanding.

Patient: *"You've been very kind, thank you for listening and being so understanding."*

Chapter 2

Why it's difficult to pass the CSA without developing fluency in patient-centredness

The wrong approach for the CSA is for the doctor to consider the patient's perspective as a specific section of the history to cover during the data gathering stage, for instance as a doctor would do for smoking history, thereby focusing mainly on the problem. The CSA is designed to assess exactly the opposite, that is, how the doctor is able to manage the patient's condition by developing a relationship with the patient to understand their unique experience.[1] The examination assesses how the doctor consults with the patient by developing the history of the problem around the patient's perspective,[2] and using this understanding to focus their further enquiry and management. The patient is encouraged to contribute throughout the consultation, to allow the views and thoughts of both parties to play a role in the partnership and decision-making, not simply add to the data.

- Works in partnership, finding common ground to develop a shared management plan.

- Develops a shared understanding with the patient.

There are three domains in the CSA:

1. **Data gathering:** the CSA assesses how the doctor **clarifies** the exact decision the patient has attended to make by encouraging the patient's contribution rather than using formulaic questions. It assesses how the doctor gathers information efficiently, taking into account the uniqueness of the patient, and tailoring their data gathering to the main task, that is, how the doctor **focuses** on the task by mainly gathering the information they need to resolve the agenda of both the patient and doctor. It is difficult to achieve this without encouraging the patient to contribute significantly during data gathering by sharing their views and thoughts. This requires rapport building and good active listening skills.

2. **Clinical management:** the CSA assesses how the doctor offers **feasible** treatment options **tailored** to the uniqueness of the patient's experience by responding to the patient's preferences and ideas. This cannot be achieved without learning how to effectively encourage the patient's contribution throughout the consultation.

3. **Interpersonal skills:** the CSA assesses how the doctor **explores** and **respond**s to the patient's perspective, understands the **impact** of the problem, puts the

problem in the context of the patient, works as a **partner** with the patient, and responds to these aspects when explaining the diagnosis and during decision-making. This cannot be achieved efficiently if the doctor is not fluent in encouraging the patient's contribution while gathering information to recognise the problem presented.

The three domains are all linked by the doctor's ability to develop a relationship with the patient within the short time frame of the encounter, using communication and consulting skills to explore the patient's experience of the problem in a way that helps the doctor to recognise the clinical problem presented and also understand the patient's experience.

In the dialogue below, the case is used to explain the grading of the CSA using the positive and negative indicators to demonstrate how the three domains are all linked to the doctor's ability to develop an understanding of the patient, regardless of the clinical problem presented, rather than focusing predominantly on the clinical problem.

The right approach

45-year-old man (152/85 mmHg last week) on 4 mg perindopril

Patient: *"The nurse asked me to attend to get my blood pressure checked."*

Opening statement.

This is the point that often shows the difference between a doctor who has practised and achieved the level of competency required to consult in a patient-centred manner and another who has rehearsed for the CSA using formulaic case-oriented books. They fail to efficiently develop an understanding of the person while gathering data for the clinical problem, and simply assume the nature of the problem the patient has attended with.

The doctor should think about the patient's perception of the situation, what they understand, how they want to proceed, and what the issue is that they would like to resolve. The doctor also needs to decide what information they need to gather from the patient to help them focus the consultation on the patient's experience in order to resolve the patient's problems and make a decision with the patient as a partner. Is the patient likely to want any treatment? What are their health beliefs? Answers to these questions should put the patient's problem in the context of the person whose health it is that the two parties are about to make a decision on. This autonomy is important in achieving patient-centredness and a shared decision. The doctor should be aware of the need to focus the consultation to the task the patient has attended to resolve, without affecting the patient's safety, by gathering data based on their knowledge of probability of the disease rather than by the use of exhaustive questioning focused mainly on the clinical problem. This aspect of keeping the consultation safe is achieved through the use of closed questions to clarify the pattern of the condition recognised by the doctor as the likely cause of the problem, while developing an understanding of the patient's experience and by excluding red flags.

Depending on the nature of the problem and the logical flow of the consultation, the doctor can also start with a clarification of the likely diagnosis and then within that context explore the patient perspective by seeking an open description of the problem by the patient. These two tasks have to be achieved efficiently by learning how to use reflective questions that are likely to encourage the patient's contribution, building a relationship with the patient based on the sharing and understanding of each other's thoughts rather than interview-type questioning.

> **Positive CSA indicators**
> - Does not use a rigid approach to consulting that fails to be sufficiently responsive to the patient's contribution.
> - Data gathering does appear to be guided by the probabilities of disease.

The doctor who accumulates information from the patient that is mainly relevant to their problem is unable to gain an understanding of the patient sufficient to focus the rest of the consultation on the exact decision the patient has attended to make. This lack of focus is the most common cause of disjointed and inefficient consultation, and poor time management.

Doctor: *"Did she say why she wanted you to get your blood pressure checked?"*

Exploring the patient's understanding. Reflective question to encourage the patient to contribute their thoughts and understanding. Avoids interruption of the patient's direction of thoughts by closing in with questions more relevant to the problem than the patient. Understands the value of perceiving the problem from the patient's perspective. Seeking to understand the patient's experience of the problem. This information gives the doctor an idea of the tasks of the consultation, the decision needing to be made, how the doctor can find a common ground for a mutual decision and the information they need to improve the explanation they will offer to the patient. Without achieving these, the doctor is unable to achieve patient-centredness.

Insufficient evidence	Needs further development	Competent	Excellent
	Develops a relationship with the patient, which works, but is focused on the problem rather than the patient.	Explores and responds to the patient's agenda, health beliefs and preferences. Elicits psychological and social information to place the patient's problem in context.	Incorporates the patient's perspective and context when negotiating the management plan.

The doctor needs to respond to the information gathered from exploring the patient's perspective of the problem, otherwise the consultation focuses on the problem rather than the patient, as described in the competency table.

Patient: *"I was a little surprised she was concerned about the blood pressure. I know it's a bit high, but that has always been the case when I rush around just before it's checked. She was in a hurry so I didn't have time to explain to her properly. She arranged some blood tests, which she said were due. I was told everything came back OK including the cholesterol. I'm in good health. I eat very healthily and exercise."*

The best way to understand how a patient feels about a problem is by encouraging their contribution to the consultation. Using a formulaic question like 'What do you think?' does not achieve the same outcome. The doctor observes the verbal cue regarding patient lifestyle.

Doctor: *"It sounds like you think the blood pressure would have been different if it was done at a different time, perhaps when you're more relaxed."*

Checking understanding. Clarifying the patient's reason for attending and the nature of the decision they have attended to make. Reflective statement with a paraphrase.

Verbal cues are useful to clarify the patient's experience and continue to encourage the patient's contribution. The doctor becomes fluent by learning the scope of the patient's experience necessary to clarify the task (the decision the patient has attended to make).

Patient: *"I keep an eye on my blood pressure at home regularly because of the nature of my job. I know for sure the tablets work because whenever I remember to take them, the blood pressure is usually around 125/80 mmHg. It can go up to 150 if I take half of the dose for instance."*

Opportunistic chance to gain insight into the social context, especially if the doctor considers it a significant aspect of the experience of the problem. Questions asked out of context are considered disjointed and unstructured because they appear illogical, and are a negative indicator in the CSA. The patient is clarifying their intentions for attending, but it's clear that at this stage the doctor is unaware of the nature of the decision. The doctor has gained an insight into the patient's train of thought and may have recognised the problem. This early recognition is important in achieving fluency and efficiency, because the skill expected from the doctor in the CSA is this recognition and their focus using this advantage in gathering data enough to clarify that recognition. A doctor who is unable to recognise the problem in this context will spend time gathering broad data around the problem to make a diagnosis and may miss the whole point of the assessment.

Insufficient evidence	Needs further development	Competent	Excellent
	Accumulates information from the patient that is mainly relevant to their problem. Uses existing information in the patient records.	Systematically gathers information, using questions appropriately targeted to the problem without affecting patient safety. Understands the importance of, and makes appropriate use of, existing information about the problem and the patient's context.	Expertly identifies the nature and scope of enquiry needed to investigate the problem, or multiple problems, within a short time-frame. Prioritises problems in a way that enhances patient satisfaction.

Doctor: *"Sounds like you vary the dose."*

Active listening. Doctor explores the patient's health beliefs. Responds to a relevant verbal cue. Exploring the patient's concerns. Using a reflective question to reassure the patient they are heard improves rapport. In the context of the blood pressure discussion, the doctor recognises the importance of understanding patient health beliefs regarding their medication and their compliance. Patients respond well to open questions that encourage their contribution.

Patient: *"My blood pressure was only picked up at work during a routine pilot medical, and at the time the doctor said it was only slightly raised. Due to the stringent rules of the pilot requirement, I was started on 4 mg perindopril just to pass the medical. I've continued taking them since, but the monthly quantity doesn't last me through the periods when I'm abroad. I cut the tablets into two, just to make sure I spread them out to last the time I'm away. I'm currently only taking 2 mg, and I suspect that may be partly why the level was raised last week. I do take my blood pressure seriously, because I wouldn't be allowed to work as a pilot if the levels are uncontrolled."*

Patient's health beliefs. Patient's unique experience of the situation, putting the problem in the context of the patient, and understanding the impact of the problem on them. Doctor clarifies the nature of the decision to be made today, and is able to focus the consultation on gathering data to help the patient resolve the problem. The doctor now understands the nature of the patient's experience. It's clearer why they felt surprised to be asked to attend, the doctor understands their thoughts about the situation and can find a common ground or a functional solution tailored to the patient's situation. This variation of management plan based on the uniqueness of the patient is what the CSA assesses and not the details of the management of medical conditions.

Positive CSA indicators
- Explores the impact of the illness on the patient's life.
- Elicits psychological and social information to place the patient's problem in context.

By using active listening and reflective questioning, the doctor is able to understand the patient's reason for the visit without making any assumptions. They are able to focus the rest of the consultation more appropriately.

Positive CSA indicator
- Clarifies the problem and nature of decision required.

Negative CSA indicator
- Makes immediate assumptions about the problem.

Doctor: *"I'll ask you specific questions to clarify your general health before we discuss the best way forward."*

The doctor uses closed questions to clarify the absence of symptoms. Checks personal and family history of heart disease (red flags), verifies working pattern and travel, smoking history, drug history/allergies, details of their lifestyle.

Signposting. Tailoring the data gathering to the problem using closed questions. Keeping the patient safe by excluding red flags. 'You didn't ask about the history of pets' is the kind of statement you might hear amongst doctors rehearsing for the examination but information should be gathered in a way to reflect the ability of the doctor to recognise a common presentation using selective enquiries to make a reasonable diagnosis based on their knowledge of likelihood while keeping the patient safe.

> *Positive CSA indicators*
> - The data gathering is guided by the probability of the disease or condition.
> - Gathers information from history taking, examination and investigation in a systematic and efficient manner.
> - Is appropriately selective in the choice of enquiries, examinations and investigations.

Doctor: *"Is it OK to examine your blood pressure and pulse?"*

Examination: BP 165/85 mmHg. Normal heart sounds and pulse.

Focused examination choices.

Doctor: *"The blood pressure is similar to the reading from last week, but I understand you're taking only 2 mg now. I know the treatment was started during a routine medical, but the levels now and when you've taken a lower amount at home, as you said, do show that your blood pressure is likely to remain high if not treated. I'm glad the tablets are helping, especially when you take the 4 mg. I think you're right about the benefit of keeping the blood pressure levels within normal, not just for your job but also for your general health. I think it's good that you're aware of the effect of your lifestyle with regards to controlling the blood pressure, but perhaps we should consider how best we can keep the level controlled most of the time."*

Doctor explains the finding, but has responded to their understanding of the patient from the way they offered that explanation. They have tailored the explanation to the uniqueness of the patient because of their understanding of the patient's views. The doctor interprets the result in context using their understanding of the patient. The doctor is seeking a common ground by giving suggestions to the patient, inviting their opinion to help them make a decision that takes into account the views of the patient in the partnership.

Insufficient evidence	Needs further development	Competent	Excellent
From the available evidence, the doctor's performance cannot be placed on a higher point of this developmental scale.	Provides explanations that are medically correct but doctor-centred.	Uses the patient's understanding to help improve the explanation offered.	Uses a variety of communication techniques and materials (e.g. written or electronic) to adapt explanations to the needs of the patient.

> *Positive CSA indicators*
> - Shows responsiveness to the patient's preferences, feelings and expectations.
> - Enhances patient autonomy.
> - Provides explanations that are relevant and understandable to the patient.

Patient: *"I think if I take the 4 mg tablets regularly, the level will be much better controlled."*

Mutual agreement and partnership in decision.

Doctor: *"Would it help if we increase the quantity of tablets you're issued with, to cover you for a longer period of time when you're not around due to your job?"*

Using their understanding of the patient's experience to offer practical, functional solutions.

Insufficient evidence	Needs further development	Competent	Excellent
	Makes decisions by applying rules, plans or protocols.	Thinks flexibly around problems generating functional solutions.	No longer relies on rules or protocols but is able to use and justify discretionary judgement in situations of uncertainty or complexity, for example in patients with multiple problems.

Patient: *"I think that would be a great idea."*

Mutual agreement.

Doctor: *"I'm happy for you to keep taking a few readings at home while you're on 4 mg, and send me a couple of these readings, perhaps in the next 2 weeks. I would expect the blood pressure levels to be much better controlled."*

Safety netting, follow-up responds to the understanding of the patient's situation. Responding to the patient's preference.

Insufficient evidence	Needs further development	Competent	Excellent
	Uses appropriate but limited management options without taking into account the preferences of the patient.	Varies management options responsively according to the circumstances, priorities and preferences of those involved.	Provides patient-centred management plans whilst taking account of local and national guidelines in a timely manner.

Patient: *"OK."*

The wrong approach

The doctor focuses on the problem and considers ICE as part of history taking.

Patient: *"The nurse asked me to attend to get my blood pressure checked."*

Doctor: *"What do you think may have caused your blood pressure to be high?"*

Formulaic, no rapport, may not encourage patient contribution. Not reflective.

Patient: *"I don't really know. As far as I know it has always been OK, apart from when it's checked immediately after I've been rushing around. I didn't explain to the nurse well last week because she was in a rush. I feel absolutely well, and eat very healthily."*

Doctor: *"How long have you been hypertensive?"*

Closed question. Focused on the problem and not the patient.

Not alert to verbal cues to develop an understanding of the patient's experience.

> **Negative CSA indicator**
> - Makes immediate assumptions about the problem.

Patient: *"Seven years."*

Doctor: *"Do you take the medication regularly?"*

Closed question. Non-reflective. Focused on the problem.

Patient: *"Yes. Occasionally when I'm running low on tablets I cut them into halves to last me till my next prescription."*

Doctor: *"Were you hoping that I could write you a new prescription?"*

Formulaic. The doctor has not demonstrated a willingness to invite the patient's views and thoughts into the conversation, and patients often react differently in these situations. They have not shared their inner feelings as they would have done if the approach was more open and inclusive. This effect (lack of rapport) is reproduced in the calibration of the CSA examination, as role players are instructed to divulge some information only when they feel the doctor has shown a genuine interest in their verbal and non-verbal expressions rather than a formulaic search for answers. The doctor does not encourage the patient's contribution sufficiently, as the approach may not be understood by the patient as an invitation to share their thoughts but rather as putting them on the spot. The question followed the patient's attempts to describe their experience and understanding of the tablets and may be seen as out of context.

> **Negative CSA indicator**
> - Uses a rigid approach to consulting that fails to be sufficiently responsive to the patient's contribution.

Patient: *"It was really the nurse who arranged the appointment. There is probably no point taking the reading today, as I'm sure it would be high. I'm only taking 2 mg of the tablets now. I would like a new prescription please."*

No relationship building, not observing verbal cues.

> **Negative CSA indicators**
> - Does not inquire sufficiently about the patient's perspective/health understanding.
> - Pays insufficient attention to the patient's verbal and non-verbal communication.

Doctor: *"Do you have any particular worries about the tablets?"*

Formulaic. Out of context. Illogical question. Makes an assumption of the problem.

Patient: *"I don't suffer any side effects at all."*

Question out of context. Patient misunderstood the intentions of the question.

Doctor:	*"What job do you do?"*

Out of context. May not encourage the building of rapport, focusing the patient on answering the doctor's questions rather than sharing their own thoughts.

Patient:	*"I'm a pilot."*
Doctor:	*"I will ask you some specific questions to clarify your general health before we discuss the best way forward."*

The doctor uses closed questions to clarify the absence of symptoms. Checks personal and family history of heart disease (red flags), verifies working pattern and travel, smoking history, drug history/allergies.

Doctor:	*"Is it OK if I check your blood pressure today?"*

Examination: BP 165/85 mmHg. Normal heart sounds and pulse.

Doctor:	*"Your blood pressure is high today. This means we need to do something to control the level."*

Not developed an understanding of the patient. Cannot empathise appropriately. Damages rapport. Explanation is offered without an understanding of the patient. No idea of the patient's views. Doctor focused on the problem. The doctor thinks their knowledge of the management of blood pressure will be assessed in detail. They cannot find a functional solution without an idea of the patient's experience of the problem.

Patient:	*"Do you mean another tablet altogether?"*

Neither party shared their thoughts. Discordance. No rapport.

Doctor:	*"I think we should increase the dose of the perindopril to 8 mg to get the levels down. Are you happy with that?"*

This is not shared decision-making. No partnership due to lack of understanding of the patient. Not encouraging the patient's contributions. Not aware of patient preferences due to lack of understanding of the patient as a person and their viewpoint.

Doctor unable to show genuine empathy due to lack of understanding of the patient's views.

Doctor showing lack of active listening.

> **Negative CSA indicator**
> - Instructs the patient rather than seeking common ground.

Patient:	*"I really don't want to increase the tablets any further if I can avoid it."*
Doctor:	*"Why's that?"*

Discordance. Poor rapport building. Discovering reason for attending late. Not aware of the main task of the consultation. Time-inefficient.

> **Negative CSA indicator**
> - Is disorganised/unsystematic in gathering information.

Patient:	*"When I take the 4 mg, the blood pressure is much better controlled. If I can have enough 4 mg to last me for a longer time, perhaps I won't need to be using 2 mg."*

Patient's preference, expectations and reason for attendance late in the consultation.

Doctor: *"I can't see any reason why we can't arrange a prescription to last you longer. May I know why you want it for longer?"*

Poor active listening. Not alert to verbal cues. Disjointed consultation. Poor time management.

Doctor: *"I'll issue a script for 2 months, is that OK?"*

Lacks understanding of the patient, and unable to put the problem into context.

Patient: *"Is it possible to make it 3 months?"*

Doctor: *"That's fine. Perhaps we can arrange a follow-up in 1 month to check the blood pressure again to make sure everything is fine, but in the meantime if you feel unwell you must let me know."*

Safety netting does not reflect an understanding of the patient's unique experience of the problem. Formulaic.

> ### Negative CSA indicators
> - Pays insufficient attention to the patient's verbal and non-verbal communication.
> - Fails to explore how the patient's life is affected by the problem.
> - Does not appreciate the impact of the patient's psychosocial context.
> - Intervenes rather than using appropriate expectant management.
> - Data gathering does not appear to be guided by the probabilities of disease.

Chapter 3

Understanding the skills assessed in the CSA

The CSA assesses the overall progress of a doctor in understanding patient-centredness, and is designed around the competencies as recommended by the RCGP.[1] These competencies can be difficult to understand in theoretical terms, and are usually best appreciated when observed and tried in real-life consultations to develop the fluency required to pass the CSA. Doctors continue to approach the examination with the wrong understanding of the competencies assessed. This situation is not helped by preparatory books which distract doctors away from the core competencies that are being assessed, directing them instead towards case-oriented preparation with the aspects of the patient's perspective as a part of a general structure rather than at the centre of the consultation. The cases presented in the CSA are designed to mimic real-life encounters to assess the application of the competencies in dealing with the problem presented by the patient in a way that shows an understanding of the patient's unique experience of that problem. This capacity to tailor the data gathering, explanation and clinical management is difficult to appreciate from case-oriented books, and role plays are unlikely to reproduce the features and uniqueness of an individual patient in real-life encounters.

In the case below, I have used an example of a typical CSA case dialogue to explore the reasons (as published by the RCGP)[1] why doctors continue to approach the examination with the wrong understanding of the competencies.

56-year-old man presenting with left hip pain

Patient: *"It's my hip again doctor."*

The opening statement gives an indication of the problem, but does not tell the doctor much about the reason for the patient's attendance. The doctor needs to understand and recognise the likely cause of the pain, and at the same time consider that the patient will need to understand the explanations they offer to them eventually. The reason for the patient's attendance cannot be assumed, as every patient is unique as to the reason they attend with a problem, or the decision they have attended to make.

The patient is also required to participate in the decision-making, so it would be difficult for the doctor to achieve a shared decision if they fail to discover the patient's own thoughts and preferences, and their experience. Therefore, a shared decision is really only achievable if there is a shared understanding of each other's thoughts. What the patient thinks about their problem may determine how they will interpret or agree with what the doctor offers, especially if that health belief is deep-seated. The best approach is for the doctor to attempt to simultaneously understand both the nature of the problem (to make a diagnosis) and the patient's experience (patient's agenda), during the data gathering phase. This means understanding and recognising the likely cause of the clinical problem through a guided exploration of the patient's own experience.

The CSA assesses how the doctor clarifies the reason for the patient's attendance, as every patient may have different intentions for and expectations from their visit; discovering these efficiently requires the use of active listening to encourage the patient to share their feelings without interruptions, so that the doctor can gain an insight into the reason for their attendance through the patient's own expression of their side of the story. This clarification is crucial in the CSA, as everything else focuses on this discovered understanding. This shared understanding is the basis of shared decision-making and the partnership relationship required to perform at a competent level in the CSA.

Positive CSA indicators
- Clarifies the problem and nature of decision required.
- Uses incremental approach, using time and accepting uncertainty.
- Gathers information efficiently, taking into account the uniqueness of the patient.
- Is selective in the choice of examination.[1]

Insufficient evidence	Needs further development	Competent	Excellent
	Accumulates information from the patient that is mainly relevant to their problem. Uses existing information in the patient records.	Systematically gathers information, using questions appropriately targeted to the problem without affecting patient safety. Understands the importance of, and makes appropriate use of, existing information about the problem and the patient's context.	Expertly identifies the nature and scope of enquiry needed to investigate the problem, or multiple problems, within a short time-frame. Prioritises problems in a way that enhances patient satisfaction.

Doctor: *"What happened exactly?"*

The doctor chose this question because he understood the value of exploring the patient's experience through their description of the problem. This question encourages the patient to share their own experience of the problem, giving the doctor an insight into why they may have attended, and possibly what they intend to achieve. It could be discovered directly or through recognition of verbal and non-verbal cues. Questions like 'Tell me about the pain' are likely to focus on the problem rather than providing an insight into the patient's interpretation, and the value of gaining this understanding will become clear through this consultation. The doctor at this stage should also be able to recognise the pattern of the problem to help them build up an impression of the likely cause. The nature of the choice of enquiry chosen depends on the opening statement of the patient, as some cases might require an initial description of the problem through the patient's perspective and some may require building the patient's thoughts and experience before the clarification of the problem, as you will observe in other chapters. If the patient has attended for a review of a test result, for instance, it may be more beneficial and efficient for the doctor to explore the patient's understanding and feelings. If, however, they had attended with a history of a dizzy spell, it may be more effective to explore the problem first, but to do this through an exploration of their experience of it. A doctor who is actively listening would be able to achieve two things here.

1. Recognise the pattern problem using knowledge of likelihood.

2. Understand the patient's experience and views.

> **Negative CSA indicator**
> - Data gathering does not appear to be guided by the probabilities of disease.

Patient: *"I've put up with it for 2 or 3 months now, but over the last 2 weeks it has just become unbearable. It catches me quite badly when I twist the left leg, and last night it was so bad that I couldn't get comfortable in bed at all."*

The doctor gains an understanding of the patient's experience and interpretation of the problem in the context of their own life. This understanding is important for the doctor to focus on the problem in such a way that they can understand how it has affected the patient's world. This insight helps the doctor understand better why they have attended.

> **Positive CSA indicator**
> - Elicits psychological and social information to place the patient's problem in context.

The context is best appreciated if the doctor learns how to encourage the patient to share their thoughts rather than asking a direct closed question about the impact, as this often can be too narrow. It is worth remembering that the impact of a problem does not necessarily have to be physical or how the doctor may have perceived it, as every individual is different.

"How bad is the pain?" is another good question that is more likely to give the doctor not only a description of the severity of the pain but a realistic chance of gaining an understanding of the impact of the problem, especially when the question is used in the context of a paraphrase to encourage the patient to share those views.

Doctor: *"It must have been quite bad last night; I wonder what could have happened in the last 2 weeks to explain the sudden change in the nature of the pain?"*

Empathy, developing patient's understanding.

This insight will improve the doctor's understanding of the nature of the decision the patient has attended to make.

Patient: *"I did a lot of walking down the seafront with my grandchildren with a bit of running the last 2 weeks, and the pain started from that point. It wasn't bad the first day, but gradually became more noticeable as the days went by. I really don't know if I've done something to it, or whether it's an entirely new problem."*

Patients share their thoughts better when the doctor shows a willingness to explore their personal experience of the problem. This approach enhances the rapport between the doctor and the patient, and gives the doctor an opportunity to genuinely empathise. The patient descriptions suggest they may have thought about the new problem, and understanding these thoughts will improve the doctor's insight into the reason for attending.

Doctor: *"It sounds like you've given some thought as to what might be causing the new pain."*

The doctor responds to the verbal cue to enhance their understanding of the patient's experience. This exploration is crucial in the CSA, and should be a way to reflect a good understanding of the patient's line of thought. This approach is learnt from practice to gain fluency and confidence in its use. The value of this approach will become clearer as the consultation unfolds.

> **Positive CSA indicators**
> - Explores patient's agenda, health beliefs and preferences.
> - Appears alert to verbal and non-verbal cues.

Patient: *"I played rugby for many years when I was younger, and sustained a lot of joint injury, especially in that same hip. I'm not sure if it's beginning to rear its head up now, but also there is a lot of arthritis in my family, which nearly crippled my mother before she passed away. Just to give you a heads-up, some of my friends at work mentioned something called bursitis. I'm hoping that's what it is, as I heard that can be treated, unlike arthritis."*

The doctor clarifies the reason for the patient's attendance, and the nature of the decision they have attended to make. They have gained an insight into the unique experience of the patient, and can put the problem in the context of the patient's life world. The most important thing is that the doctor now understands the problem from the patient's perspective, and is in a position to work with the patient as a true partner to help the patient make the best decision for them. It is important to understand that this consultation is not about a 'hip pain' but 'Mr Smith's hip pain', and this is what Mr Smith really wants the doctor to help him with. The doctor has their own agenda, which is to recognise the likely cause of the problem after excluding other potential alternative causes, and to suggest the best way forward using their knowledge tailored to the patient. This is what the CSA assesses.

Doctor: *"It sounds like this has really bothered you."*

The doctor, through active listening, understands the need to clarify the nature of the impact of the problem from the patient's perspective. He has responded to a verbal cue from the patient's thoughts and feelings about the situation. He has chosen a question likely to allow the patient to share their views on the situation, both in terms of their thoughts about it and its physical impact.

Insufficient evidence	Needs further development	Competent	Excellent
From the available evidence, the doctor's performance cannot be placed on a higher point of this developmental scale.	Recognises the impact of the problem on the patient.	Recognises the impact of the problem on the patient, their family and/or carers.	Recognises and shows understanding of the limits of the doctor's ability to intervene in the holistic care of the patient.

> **Positive CSA indicators**
> - Explores the impact of the illness on the patient's life.
> - Elicits psychological and social information to place the patient's problem in context.

Patient: *"I know arthritis can get in the way of life, as I saw it happen to my mother. I do a lot of model work in my garage which involves a lot of standing, and I can't imagine not being able to do that if this turns out to be arthritis. Going upstairs is becoming a bit of problem as well."*

The patient's concerns are best appreciated from allowing the patient – through reflective guidance – to share their experience, as within that context the doctor is likely to gain insight. It is not uncommon for a patient's concern to be the reason for their attendance or vice versa. Formulaic questions are often less rewarding as they do not follow a logical pattern when asked as a part of a conventional history in an exhaustive manner.

The best way to understand the severity of a problem is to explore the impact of the problem from the patient's perspective. The value of this understanding is seen during the stage of decision-making, as the doctor is likely to respond to that understanding in the tailoring of their advice. This understanding is also important for offering explanations to the patient to improve their understanding.

> **Positive CSA indicators**
> - Explores the patient's agenda, health beliefs and preferences.
> - Appears alert to verbal and non-verbal cues.

Doctor: *"I'm now going to ask you some specific questions to help me understand the pain a bit better."*

Signposting. The CSA assesses how a doctor is able to use closed questions to clarify their recognition of a common presentation. The question needs to be very selective, and should have a realistic aim. In this case the doctor thinks about a possible osteoarthritis, perhaps trochanteric bursitis, tendon causes, radiculopathies, and sinister causes in general. The question the doctor needs to ask in order to exclude any of the above conditions should be very targeted, especially with regards to the possibility of bursitis, and should respond to their understanding of the patient.

The patient describes pain that is worse on lying on the same side, and not painful on just standing. There is no redness or swelling or back pain and they feel well, and haven't lost any weight.

> **Positive CSA indicators**
> - Is selective in the choice of examination.
> - Gathers information efficiently, taking into account the uniqueness of the patient.
> - Data gathering appears to be guided by the probabilities of disease.
> - Is appropriately selective in the choice of enquiries, examinations and investigations.

Insufficient evidence	Needs further development	Competent	Excellent
	Accumulates information from the patient that is mainly relevant to their problem. Uses existing information in the patient records.	Systematically gathers information, using questions appropriately targeted to the problem without affecting patient safety. Understands the importance of, and makes appropriate use of, existing information about the problem and the patient's context.	Expertly identifies the nature and scope of enquiry needed to investigate the problem, or multiple problems, within a short time-frame. Prioritises problems in a way that enhances patient satisfaction.

Doctor: *"Would it be OK if I had a look at the hip for you, to see if I can work out what would be the most likely cause?"*

Examination: normal passive and active movement of the hip. Localised tenderness over the greater trochanter.

Insufficient evidence	Needs further development	Competent	Excellent
	Chooses examination broadly in line with the patient's problem(s).	Chooses examinations appropriately targeted to the patient's problem(s).	Proficiently identifies and performs the scope of examination necessary to investigate the patient's problem(s).

Positive CSA indicator
- Is appropriately selective in the choice of enquiries, examinations and investigations.

Doctor: *"Your hip moves very well without causing you any pain, but you do have a soreness just over the area on the outside of the hip when I pressed on it. This is exactly the area where the hip joint has a small pocket called a bursa. It's possible that this bursa is inflamed, as your friend had mentioned. This is why you had a lot of pain when you were lying on that same side, and also why you struggled mostly with the stairs and twisting the leg. I don't think the main problem is arthritis, otherwise it would have been painful when I moved the hip during the examination, possibly explaining why you're more comfortable when you're up and about or standing. I don't think it would have been as a result of injuries from rugby, but perhaps the walking and running you've been doing recently didn't help."*

The doctor responds to their understanding of the patient's perspective and experience of the problem by using an explanation that demonstrates that understanding. The patient is likely to relate to the explanation, as it directly explains their unique experience of the problem. If the doctor did not gain this understanding in the initial phases, it would have been difficult to enhance the explanation they offer to the patient. The doctor also demonstrated from the explanation that they understood the patient's reasons for attending, and the nature of the decision they have attended to make. The doctor understands how important it is for the patient to know they haven't got arthritis, and is able to allay that fear. This is exactly what the CSA is designed to assess.

Insufficient evidence	Needs further development	Competent	Excellent
From the available evidence, the doctor's performance cannot be placed on a higher point of this developmental scale.	Provides explanations that are medically correct but doctor-centred.	Uses the patient's understanding to help improve the explanation offered.	Uses a variety of communication techniques and materials (e.g. written or electronic) to adapt explanations to the needs of the patient.

Positive CSA indicators
- Places the problem in the perspective of the uniqueness of the patient.
- Shows responsiveness to the patient's feelings, preferences and expectations.
- Provides explanations that are relevant to the patient.
- Responds to patient's concerns with interest.

Patient: *"I'm so relieved to hear it isn't arthritis, as the thoughts overwhelmed me last night. I couldn't stop thinking about how I may have to give up my hobby of car modelling."*

Patient's concerns addressed. Task achieved through partnership.

Doctor: *"You were right about the bursitis being treatable. I'm not sure exactly what you're currently taking for the pain."*

Finding a common ground. Checking understanding.

- Uses an incremental approach, using time and accepting uncertainty.

Patient: *"I used some anti-inflammatory tablets, which have helped a bit. I don't think I will need any more painkillers, to be honest, as I'm managing OK."*

Negotiation. Mutual agreement. Partnership. Offers are tailored to the patient.

Positive CSA indicators
- Offers appropriate and feasible management options.
- Works in partnership and finds common ground.

Doctor: *"This condition can sometimes actually resolve on its own, but there are a few things we can do to help it get better. It's important to avoid lying on that side if you can, as putting pressure on it won't help it get better. You can apply some cold compress over the area when it's quite bad to relieve the discomfort, as it does help with the inflammation as well. I know the stairs have been a bit of a problem, how are you going to cope with that?"*

Thinking flexibly around a problem to find functional and practical solutions.

Using time as a tool.

Understanding the principle of watch and wait.

Empowering the patient.

Insufficient evidence	Needs further development	Competent	Excellent
	Makes decisions by applying rules, plans or protocols.	Thinks flexibly around problems generating functional solutions.	No longer relies on rules or protocols but is able to use and justify discretionary judgement in situations of uncertainty or complexity, for example in patients with multiple problems.

> *Positive CSA indicator*
> - Uses an incremental approach, using time and accepting uncertainty.

Patient: *"I spend most of my daytime downstairs anyway, so it shouldn't really be a problem. I may have to find a chair to sit on when I'm working in the garage with my models."*

Mutual agreement. Partnership.

Doctor: *"I think that sounds reasonable. We recommend a bit of stretching exercise every now and then, but I'll give you a sheet that will guide you about how often and when."*

Incremental approach to offering advice.

Seeking agreement and common ground.

Insufficient evidence	Needs further development	Competent	Excellent
	Suggests intervention in all cases.	Considers a "wait and see" approach where appropriate. Uses effective prioritisation of problems when the patient presents with multiple issues.	Empowers the patient with confidence to manage problems independently together with knowledge of when to seek further help.

Doctor: *"Normally I would expect – perhaps in the next 2–4 weeks – for things to improve for you, but if it persists or gets any worse we could meet again and discuss other options that might help you with the problem."*

Safety net should reflect a reasonable understanding of the natural course of the condition.

It should be relevant and feasible to the patient, showing the doctor's understanding of the patient's experience.

Demonstrates the doctor's understanding of foreseeable risks.

Patient: *"That's fine; I'll let you know how I get on."*

Chapter 4

How to understand the patient's perspective without using formulaic questions

This book uses an approach which encourages the doctor to discover the reasons for the patient's attendance and the nature of the issue they want help resolving, avoiding the use of formulaic pre-prepared questions. The aim is to clarify the patient's ideas, concerns and expectations using reflective questioning and active listening to develop an understanding of the patient's perspective. The patient's ideas and expectations are usually part of their interpretation of their problem, and understanding this perspective helps the doctor to gain an insight into the patient's life, and to focus the rest of the enquiry on the main issues that are important and relevant to the patient, giving the consultation a logical flow rather than a disjointed approach. If this focus on the patient agenda is not achieved, the consultation is unlikely to achieve the task in partnership with the patient, causing discordance in the later stages of the consultation. In the dialogue below, the doctor uses information from the patient to effectively build up a picture of the patient's perspective. This gives the doctor an idea of the scope of enquiries to use, and the nature of the decision both parties are to make together.

58-year-old woman

Patient: *"I've had problems with my ankle for a long time on and off, but although the ankle has been better over the last few months, my left knee has started giving me a lot of problems. It feels stiff after I have sat down or not used it for a while, and causes me a lot of problems going up stairs. The pain is mostly at the sides of the knee but the position of the pain varies from day to day. I'm not really sure what to make of it, but have decided to get someone to have a look at it."*

The patient opening statement gives the doctor a general idea of the scope of the problem, but doesn't yet make clear the patient's experience of the problem. At this stage the doctor should not be distracted by the clinical diagnosis but should mainly focus on understanding the patient's experience and trying to recognise the most likely cause of the problem from the patient's descriptions. The doctor needs to consider what might be going on in the mind of the patient, and they can do this effectively by using reflective questioning to encourage the patient to share those views further. Focusing on the clinical problem at this stage may not give the doctor a sufficient understanding of the patient's experience, or the level of focus required to achieve a systematic data gathering.

> **Positive CSA indicators**
> - Gathers information from history taking, examination and investigation in a systematic and efficient manner.
> - Is appropriately selective in the choice of enquiries, examinations and investigations.

Doctor: *"It sounds like you've been trying to work out what might have brought the pain on."*

Reflective question based on an understanding of the direction of thoughts of the patient, aimed at encouraging further contribution from the patient to gain an understanding of what and how the patient feels about the problem.

> **Positive CSA indicators**
> - Explores the patient's agenda, health beliefs and preferences.
> - Appears alert to verbal and non-verbal cues.

Patient: *"I really don't know, but I do have some varicose veins in both legs, and perhaps it could be that they're part of the problem. I'm planning to visit my daughter in Australia in two weeks and wasn't sure if I would be able to go, as you hear all sorts of problems about clots on the plane. I can't remember hurting myself either, although I did a long walk in Cornwall just a few weeks before the pain got worse. One does wonder sometimes of course whether something like this could just be due to age, although I wouldn't have expected it to be sudden like this."*

This information puts the patient's problem in context, and gives the doctor an opportunity to work in partnership with the patient using this understanding. The information the patient has provided gives the doctor an opportunity to understand the patient's perspective of the problem, improving the doctor's insight into the patient's reasons for attending. The doctor still needs to clarify the nature of the clinical problem, and understand the nature of the decision both parties are going to make.

- Explores the patient's agenda, health beliefs and preferences.

- Appears alert to verbal and non-verbal cues.

Doctor: *"I can see you've really thought about it. Can you tell me how bad it has really been for you?"*

This question was chosen to gain an insight into the severity of the problem from the patient's point of view, which gives the doctor an idea of the impact of the problem on the patient, and is likely to put the problem in the right context. This is different from using a formulaic question like "How has it affected your job?" which is too closed and narrow.

Patient: *"I don't have any pains today, but on some days the pain can be really bad. I struggle mostly with bending forward to pick things up from the floor, and it worries me how I'm going to cope in Australia with running after my granddaughter and picking her up. The most difficult is when I climb stairs, but I can walk OK on a flat surface. I've been frightened of doing anything specifically to it so that I wouldn't make it worse, but now I think I need to understand exactly what may be the cause to help me know how to handle it."*

Positive CSA indicators
- Explores the impact of the illness on the patient's life.
- Elicits psychological and social information to place the patient's problem in context.

Doctor: *"I can understand why you've been concerned about the pains. What have you been doing so far to help?"*

Empathy, finding a common ground to help in sharing the decision using the doctor's ability to recognise the problem from the descriptions given so far. This use of the understanding of the probability of the disease based on prevalence is a useful skill to help the doctor focus the consultation to the task rather than using an exhaustive line of enquiries to make a diagnosis.

Negative CSA indicators
- Is disorganised/unsystematic in gathering information.
- Data gathering does not appear to be guided by the probabilities of disease.

Patient: *"I've only taken some paracetamol, which has helped, but I've been afraid to take anything else stronger because of the blood pressure tablets I take. I've even rubbed some cream I bought in the chemist over the area, which has also helped, but what concerns me most is to make sure I know exactly what is causing the pain rather than just covering it up with painkillers."*

The patient feels encouraged to participate in the consultation due to the nature of the doctor's approach. They're able to share their views, giving the doctor an idea of the reasons for their attendance. The doctor is now able to focus the rest of the consultation efficiently using the understanding they have gained of the patient's perspective. This cannot be achieved if the focus of the consultation is mainly on the clinical problem. It is important for the doctor to develop an ability to recognise a common clinical problem in this way, and then use closed questions later on to clarify their own agenda more efficiently without affecting the patient's safety.

Positive CSA indicators
- Clarifies the problem and nature of the decision required.
- Uses an incremental approach, using time and accepting uncertainty.

Doctor: *"Would you be able to describe the pain that you're getting?"*

Patient: *"I've always had twinges in both knees, but this one catches me when I try to get up from sitting, for instance. There hasn't been any swelling or anything, but the pain can be a bit annoying at night in bed. On some days I don't have any pains at all. I can walk OK most of the time, but I feel the soreness when I press on the inside of the knee sometimes."*

The doctor understands and recognises the possible cause of the problem from the description given by the patient of a common presentation, but would need to use their knowledge of probabilities to confirm the diagnosis and exclude other serious alternative causes.

Positive CSA indicators
- Recognises presentations of common physical, psychological and social problems.
- Data gathering appears to be guided by the probabilities of disease.

Doctor: *"I'm going to ask you some specific questions to help me understand the problem a bit better."*

The doctor uses a closed question to confirm their suspicion of a possible flare-up of osteoarthritis. They exclude significant intra-articular causes using questions to confirm absence of locking or the leg giving way. They verify the absence of systemic symptoms, and exclude red flags like redness and swelling. They clarify the drug history, and allergies.

> **Positive CSA indicator**
> - Is appropriately selective in the choice of enquiries, examinations and investigations.

Doctor: *"Is it OK if I have a good look at the knee?"*

Examination: mild osteoarthritis.

Doctor: *"From the examination, it does seem that the main pain is coming from the joint itself, and I felt a little creaking when I moved it. This often represents a possible 'wear and tear' from within the joints. The area where you have the varicose veins doesn't look inflamed, and is very unlikely to be the cause of the pain. I know you were wondering about how quickly the pain has come on, but sometimes that can happen when the joint is jarred a bit, perhaps from the long walk in Cornwall, but there are no signs suggesting that you won't be able to travel to Australia."*

The doctor uses their understanding of the patient to improve the information they offer them to enhance the patient's understanding of the explanation. This is different from just using non-medical jargon, but the doctor is showing their responsiveness to the patient's perspectives.

> **Positive CSA indicators**
> - Shows responsiveness to the patient's preferences, feelings and expectations.
> - Enhances patient autonomy.
> - Provides explanations that are relevant and understandable to the patient.

Patient: *"I didn't know you could have wear and tear in the joint without having pains until it flares. That would make a lot of sense."*

Shared understanding.

Doctor: *"I know you were mostly concerned about how you would cope with your trip to Australia regarding getting around. When the wear and tear flares up like this, often it does settle again but you may find that painkillers make things a little bit easier for you. I know you've tried paracetamol, but you can certainly take painkillers stronger than paracetamol safely in combination with your blood pressure tablets – perhaps you could consider taking something like that on days when the pain is too bad."*

Offering advice showing an understanding of the uniqueness of the patient's experience.

> **Positive CSA indicators**
> - Offers appropriate and feasible management options.
> - Shows responsiveness to the patient's preferences, feelings and expectations.
> - Responds to needs and concerns with interest and understanding.
> - Is cooperative and inclusive in approach.

Patient: *"I will definitely find those helpful for now and hope that the pain will ease."*

Shared understanding and shared decision.

> **Positive CSA indicator**
> - Works in partnership, finding common ground to develop a shared management plan.

Doctor: *"It will also be helpful to continue to do gentle exercises of the knee as much as the pain will let you, to keep the joint moving and stop it getting stiff. It's best to avoid any strenuous movements that will aggravate the pain in the meantime. I'm not sure how you feel about that?"*

Suggesting treatment option, and not instructive.

> **Positive CSA indicators**
> - Works in partnership, finding common ground to develop a shared management plan.
> - Encourages improvement, rehabilitation, and, where appropriate, recovery.
> - Encourages the patient to participate in appropriate health promotion and disease prevention strategies.

Patient: *"I'll certainly continue moving the joint and perhaps the painkillers will come in handy."*

Patient empowered to play a role in decision-making.

Doctor: *"Normally I would expect the pain to ease within the next couple of weeks, but assuming you start feeling the pains even more or you notice that you're struggling to bear your weight – especially if you notice your legs giving way – then you must let me know so we can reconsider our plan."*

Showing an understanding of uncertainties.

> **Positive CSA indicators**
> - Makes plans that reflect the natural history of common problems.
> - Manages risk effectively, safety netting appropriately.
> - Uses an incremental approach, using time and accepting uncertainty.

Patient: *"I will definitely let you know how I get on."*

Chapter 5

Achieving patient-centredness regardless of the nature of the clinical problem

Often in the examination and in real life, patients attend to discuss results of tests. It is difficult sometimes to know the amount of information required to be discussed in these consultations within the limited amount of time, to maximise the opportunity presented by the consultation to educate and empower the patient. The same approach as used in this book will achieve the right balance of information using patient-centredness. The information offered to the patient should reflect the doctor's understanding of the patient, highlighting the importance of approaching the consultation with the patient's experience at the centre of the data gathering, regardless of the nature of the clinical condition.

Doctors rehearse how to discuss medical conditions with patients by practising the use of non-medical jargon, but according to the competency tested in the CSA, the explanation should be tailored to the individual patient by offering advice or information which reflects the doctor's understanding of that particular patient. This means that the patient may not necessarily understand a medically correct non-jargon explanation of a result or condition as well as they would have done if the explanation was offered in a way that reflected the doctor's understanding of the patient's own thoughts, thereby improving their understanding.

The dialogue below demonstrates how patient-centredness can be applied in any consultation, as the explanation of a condition or a test can be the first opportunity for the doctor to **'respond'** to their understanding of the patient. The competency table below clearly shows that the doctor is required to not only explore the patient's experience and understanding, but also respond to that understanding.

Insufficient evidence	Needs further development	Competent	Excellent
	Develops a relationship with the patient, which works, but is focused on the problem rather than the patient.	Explores and responds to the patient's agenda, health beliefs and preferences. Elicits psychological and social information to place the patient's problem in context.	Incorporates the patient's perspective and context when negotiating the management plan.

23-year-old woman (B$_{12}$ 75; pernicious anaemia screen negative; HB 14)

Patient: *"I had a blood test last week, and I've come to discuss the results."*

Opening statement. Gives the doctor an indication of the nature of the task ahead, but often not enough for the doctor to clarify the outcome the patient wants or the reason for the patient's attendance. The doctor actively listens with a view to understanding the patient's experience of the situation so far. The doctor explores the patient's understanding of what has happened through the patient's perspective. This will enable the doctor to gain more insight into the reason for the patient's attendance, their thoughts about the situation, their preferences and maybe their concerns. These may require clarification by observing verbal cues carefully or exploring the thoughts of the patient through active listening. Reflective questions are useful in encouraging the patient's contribution and achieving the above. If the doctor chooses a follow-up question which is centred on the problem, they are unlikely to encourage the patient's contribution in a way that will help them understand the thoughts and feelings of the patient.

A negative indicator in the CSA is when a doctor immediately assumes the patient's reason for attending, without attempting to develop that insight through an understanding of the patient's experience. This insight could be developed by choosing a line of enquiry that reassures the patient that they were heard.

Negative CSA indicator
- Makes immediate assumptions about the problem.

The doctor should consider an open question to demonstrate that they listened and understood what the patient has said, and to encourage the patient to continue to tell their story and share their thoughts. This systematic way of gathering information is likely to increase the doctor's insight into the exact reason for the patient's attendance, so the doctor will be able to focus on the exact task the patient has attended to discuss rather than a broad non-systematic search for a diagnosis.

In this dialogue it's possible the patient could have a different understanding of the reason for the blood test, or may have other views with regards to the test and its interpretation. Establishing these views puts the visit in context, giving the doctor an idea of the nature of the decision the patient may have attended to make.

From the table below, it is clear that accumulating information from the patient that is mainly relevant to the patient's problems, rather than the patient as a whole, is a negative indicator in the CSA. Using patient-centred consultation techniques every day will help the doctor to identify the nature and scope of enquiry needed to clarify the reason for the patient's attendance, and understand the patient as whole more efficiently, within a shorter time frame.[4]

Insufficient evidence	Needs further development	Competent	Excellent
	Accumulates information from the patient that is mainly relevant to their problem. Uses existing information in the patient records.	Systematically gathers information, using questions appropriately targeted to the problem without affecting patient safety. Understands the importance of, and makes appropriate use of, existing information about the problem and the patient's context.	Expertly identifies the nature and scope of enquiry needed to investigate the problem, or multiple problems, within a short time-frame. Prioritises problems in a way that enhances patient satisfaction.

Doctors who are not able to approach the consultation in a way that initially gives the patient an opportunity to participate in the consultation through sharing their views are likely to focus more on the clinical problem and will not show responsiveness to the patient.

> **Positive CSA indicators**
> - Is appropriately selective in the choice of enquiries, examinations and investigations.
> - Shows responsiveness to the patient's preferences, feelings and expectations.

Doctor: *"Can you tell me what you understand so far regarding the tests that you had done?"*

Reflective question. Encouraging patient's contribution. Getting the patient's perspective. Clarifying the reason for attending and the nature of the task for the consultation. The doctor chose this question because they want to understand the patient and what they have made of previous consultations and possibly their current thoughts about the situation.

> **Positive CSA indicators**
> - Explores the patient's agenda, health beliefs and preferences.
> - Appears alert to verbal and non-verbal cues.

Patient: *"I had several small ulcers in the mouth over the last few months and the doctor recommended that I have a blood test. The result came back that I was low on B_{12}, but he arranged for a special test to check if I was anaemic. I have had anaemia before, when I had to take iron tablets, so it won't surprise me if I am anaemic. I really don't know why I would have been low on iron, as I eat healthily and I'm not a vegetarian. I feel well in myself but I guess it's probably only just become low, so I wouldn't have felt the symptoms of anaemia as yet."*

Patient's thoughts. Insight into reason for attending. Patient's unique experience. The patient's thoughts are important in the partnership, as the information the doctor offers later on should be based on their understanding of the patient's views. The patient's concerns and thoughts will guide the doctor to use this understanding to focus their data gathering. Without this information, the doctor is unlikely to be selective with their choice of enquiry, lacking a systematic approach to data gathering.

> **Positive CSA indicators**
> - Clarifies the problem and nature of decision required.
> - Gathers information efficiently, taking into account the uniqueness of the patient.
> - Is selective in the choice of examination.

Doctor: *"You seem to know a little bit about the B_{12}."*

Responding to verbal cues.

Reflective question. Actively listening to gain an understanding of the patient's beliefs and thoughts. Preparing a common ground for the decision to be made later. In the CSA the doctor is expected to recognise common problems that present to general practice through their experience in day-to-day practice. The doctor recognises the patient has been thinking about the possible problem here and is trying to understand the patient's level of knowledge, which will help the doctor provide information in a way the patient will understand better.

Patient: *"I have read up on it. I know you can get a lot of B_{12} in red meat and liver, but these are foods I don't particularly like and so don't eat them often. I do eat a lot of Greek yoghurt and that contains about 0.7 µg of B_{12} per pot. I don't have any dietary restrictions. I don't have any problems with my bowel movements or anything, and haven't noticed any of the symptoms mentioned on the NHS website."*

The doctor can only achieve an organised and structured consultation if they are able to recognise the tasks the patient has attended to deal with. This is very useful as it allows the doctor to follow a logical approach in data gathering, and to achieve an outcome which is meaningful and relevant to the patient. Otherwise the approach is likely to involve a broad questioning, which often does not address the issues that are important to the patient.

Insufficient evidence	Needs further development	Competent	Excellent
	Consults to an acceptable standard but lacks focus and requires longer consulting times.	Consults in an organised and structured way, achieving the main tasks of the consultation in a timely manner.	Consults effectively in a focused manner, moving beyond the essential to take a holistic view of the patient's needs within the time-frame of a normal consultation.

Positive CSA indicators
- Gathers information from history taking, examination and investigation in a systematic and efficient manner.
- Is appropriately selective in the choice of enquiries, examinations and investigations.

Doctor: *"I can see you've gained a lot of useful knowledge about B_{12}. Sounds like you are concerned you may not be getting enough through your diet."*

Responding to relevant cue which helps this doctor prepare for the advice they may offer.

The doctor is now focusing on gathering data that are relevant to the reason the patient has attended. The consultation is focused on the exact nature of the decision the patient has attended to make. A common mistake is trying to be broad with the line of questioning so as to cover every possibility, but the competency grading expects the doctor to recognise a common problem presented within the context of the patient's description using their knowledge of likelihood.

Positive CSA indicators
- Is appropriately selective in the choice of enquiries, examinations and investigations.
- Data gathering appears to be guided by the probabilities of disease.

Patient: *"I was a little concerned when I had a look online at the first 20 food items high in B_{12}, as it's only salmon that I enjoy eating on the list. I'm not sure, if I'm going to replace the vitamin B_{12} by diet, which food really would be the best for me, but the website did mention about some horrible complications of B_{12} deficiency."*

Patient's thoughts and concerns. Patient feels encouraged to share her views. The doctor is building partnership and rapport, and able to genuinely empathise with the patient. The problem is put in the context of the patient.

Insufficient evidence	Needs further development	Competent	Excellent
	Develops a relationship with the patient, which works, but is focused on the problem rather than the patient.	Explores and responds to the patient's agenda, health beliefs and preferences. Elicits psychological and social information to place the patient's problem in context.	Incorporates the patient's perspective and context when negotiating the management plan.

Doctor: *"I'm going to ask you some specific questions to help me understand the situation a bit better."*

Signposting. The doctor uses a closed question to clarify the absence of symptoms of anaemia and neuropathy. The doctor excludes any systemic illness and weight loss. Red flags. Family history, drug history and allergies. Clarifies any history of blood loss or bowel changes.

This is a section many doctors spend most of their preparation on. It's not surprising that this is not an area considered to be one of the most common reasons for failure, as most doctors would have gained enough knowledge and experience to identify common medical conditions that present in general practice. The problem here is that the CSA assesses how the doctor then applies their experience in tailoring their knowledge to the individual patient. The doctor has a very limited time to explore the condition in its entirety but should have enough time to explore aspects of the condition enough to help the patient with the task they have attended with, and then using red flags to keep the patient safe. A common mistake is when the doctor does not develop this ability to recognise the pattern of the clinical problem using their knowledge of likelihood. They should then ask questions that demonstrate a logical way of thinking to clarify their own thoughts about the problem and exclude other causes using effective closed questions. It is important to remember that the competency recommended is an incremental approach to diagnosis, showing an ability to use time as a tool, and effective use of red flags and safety nets to maintain patient safety.

> **Positive CSA indicators**
> - Recognises presentation of common problem.
> - Uses incremental approach, using time and accepting uncertainty.
> - Is selective in the choice of examination.
> - Gathers information efficiently, taking into account the uniqueness of the patient.

Doctor: *"I will have a look at your eyes and your blood pressure to make sure there are no obvious signs of anaemia."*

Examination: no pallor. BP 123/80, pulse 70/min.

The choice of examination to reflect a doctor's logical understanding of what is needed to resolve the decision the patient has attended to make and maintain patient safety. It should be very focused on the tasks to resolve both the patient's and the doctor's agenda.

Doctor: *"You're right about the vitamin B_{12} being low. I know you were concerned about anaemia. The blood levels are kept normal as long as the body is making the blood, but the problem is that the body needs the B_{12} to help make the blood. If the levels remain too low, then it gets to a point where the body will not have enough B_{12}. That is the point when the person may become anaemic. You are not anaemic now, as you suspected, but we need to discuss how we can replace the B_{12} to avoid the possibility of developing anaemia. I know the second test was for pernicious anaemia. That doesn't mean the doctor thought you were anaemic, but we know that occasionally people are born with a condition where they are not able to absorb the B_{12} even though they have a lot of it in their food. That is what the second test was for, but your result shows that you do not have that condition. I would then expect that if you were to increase your intake of food containing B_{12}, we should notice some improvements in the level, avoiding the possibilities of anaemia or the complication that you mentioned. I'm not sure if you understand."*

The doctor explains the result and the situation using their appreciation of the patient's understanding of the situation. This doesn't mean just avoiding medical jargon but using the language that reflects the doctor's understanding of the patient's views, preferences and concerns to improve the explanation offered.

Insufficient evidence	Needs further development	Competent	Excellent
From the available evidence, the doctor's performance cannot be placed on a higher point of this developmental scale.	Provides explanations that are medically correct but doctor-centred.	Uses the patient's understanding to help improve the explanation offered.	Uses a variety of communication techniques and materials (e.g. written or electronic) to adapt explanations to the needs of the patient.

Some doctors prepare for this section of the consultation in a formulaic manner, learning how to explain medical diagnosis to a patient with non-medical jargon. Although it is right not to use jargon, what is more important is to use the patient's understanding to help improve the explanation. This is a crucial part of the consultation, which gives the doctor an opportunity to **'respond'** and show their understanding of the patient. Telling a patient that their sore throat was caused by a virus instead of bacteria is medically correct useful information, but what might be more useful is to explain to them using the doctor's understanding of their experience and views. For example, 'Your sore throat is not the type that requires antibiotics to get better, and is very unlikely to cause problems with your new tooth'. This second explanation has taken into account the patient's concerns about their new tooth getting infected as a result of the sore throat, and also directly addressed their request for information about whether the sore throat will need antibiotics. The doctor can then explain, if necessary, the differences between bacteria and viruses, depending on their understanding of their patient.

Patient: *"I see. I'm not anaemic yet, so replacing the B_{12} will prevent that from happening. Considering the complications that can happen, I should try as hard as possible to include more foods that are high in B_{12} into my diet, and see how much the levels will rise."*

Patient's contribution. This is why a shared agreement is referred to as a partnership. The patient's preferences do not have to be taken as the best plan, but should be taken into consideration during the decision-making. The patient understands the information offered to them better when that information has been made relevant to their unique situation, which empowers the patient further.

Doctor: *"I know you had iron tablets in the past, but this situation is different from iron deficiency. One can become anaemic from lack of iron in just the same way as lack of B_{12}, but they are different nutrients for blood making."*

The doctor is able to clarify this information to the patient as a result of their understanding of the patient's health beliefs. This way of giving information empowers the patient and is likely to be understood. The relevance of the information offered to the patient is essential in the CSA grading.

> **Positive CSA indicators**
> - Provides explanations that are relevant and understandable to the patient.
> - Enhances patient autonomy.
> - Works in partnership, finding common ground to develop a shared management plan.

Doctor: *"I know you don't like most of the food you looked at online, but I'll give you a detailed list of food items to check if you can find more options to choose from, but you have to bear in mind that some of the food items may contain much larger quantities of B_{12} than others. There is also an option of tablets that contain B_{12}, which we can use to supplement your efforts, at least in the meantime. These tablets are more likely to guarantee that you're getting a definite amount of B_{12}, at least while you're still experimenting with the best way to change your diet."*

Offering options in an incremental manner. Seeking the patient's agreement and opinion.

The CSA assesses the ability of the doctor to tailor the advice given to the patient, and also to think flexibly around a problem to find practical and functional solutions. This ability to vary the management plan cannot be achieved without approaching the consultation with a view to making the patient's perspective a central source of information, otherwise there is a chance the doctor then offers all the possible options without tailoring the option to suit the patient's own unique situation and preferences.

The dietitian service can be a useful option to offer, if it is available locally.

Insufficient evidence	Needs further development	Competent	Excellent
	Uses appropriate but limited management options without taking into account the preferences of the patient.	Varies management options responsively according to the circumstances, priorities and preferences of those involved.	Provides patient-centred management plans whilst taking account of local and national guidelines in a timely manner.
	Makes decisions by applying rules, plans or protocols.	Thinks flexibly around problems generating functional solutions.	No longer relies on rules or protocols but is able to use and justify discretionary judgement in situations of uncertainty or complexity, for example in patients with multiple problems.

Patient: *"I would prefer to try the diet first and see what I can manage, as I'd prefer not to take tablets unless I really can't get a good intake from my diet."*

Patient's preferences. Patient feels encouraged to share their views. Patient plays a role in the decision-making due to nature of the options offered to them by the doctor. The decision can only be considered to be shared if all the parties in the partnership are able to share their thoughts about any option. This can be time-consuming if not rehearsed very well in real life, but practising how to use an incremental approach to management is what the CSA assesses. It is in fact preferable to run out of time in the CSA whilst offering management to a patient in an incremental manner which responds to their preferences, rather than rushing through a list of management options for that condition without working through the options in partnership with the patient. This approach scores very low in interpersonal skills, and the doctor will appear very formulaic.

Doctor: *"That sounds reasonable; perhaps it would be a good idea for us to check the levels again in about 3 months to see what you've achieved with diet. Maybe at that time, we can consider using the supplement if the levels remain low. In the meantime, if you notice that you're beginning to feel tired or unwell, you must let me know, although I won't expect the blood anaemia to change significantly within that timeframe."*

Mutually agreed plan. Relevant safety netting tailored to address the patient's concern, reflecting the doctor's understanding of the patient's feelings and concerns. Doctor uses their knowledge of the natural course of the condition to manage the risk presented by the patient's preference. This knowledge of risk is best demonstrated through the use of red flag closed questions and the nature of follow-up arrangement the doctor puts in place to demonstrate the patient's safety.

Positive CSA indicators
- Makes plans that reflect the natural history of common problems.
- Management approaches reflect an appropriate assessment of risk.
- Manages risk effectively, safety netting appropriately.
- Works in partnership, finding common ground to develop a shared management plan.
- Shows responsiveness to the patient's preferences, feelings and expectations.
- Enhances patient autonomy.

Patient: *"OK, thanks."*

Chapter 6

The patient's understanding and experience

The impression that developing the patient's understanding makes a consultation take longer is common,[3] but the opposite is the case when the doctor achieves the fluency and understanding of the skills required to achieve the focus needed for patient-centredness. The problem often arises when the doctor is not aware when they have explored the patient's perspective sufficiently. The value of gaining an insight into the patient's perspective is beneficial at all stages of the consultation, ranging from clarifying the reason for the patient's attendance, clarifying the decision needed to be made (task), recognising the problem, focusing the data gathering, focusing the choice of examination, improving the explanation offered, varying the options, sharing decisions, finding common ground, finding a practical solution to the patient's problem, and safety netting appropriately. These are the key areas assessed in the CSA, in particular how much the doctor has developed the flexibility to use this approach regardless of the level of knowledge they may or may not have about the clinical condition. It is clear from the above how the three domains in the CSA depend on the doctor's ability to build a therapeutic relationship with the patient through an understanding of the patient's experience.

In the consultation, the patient's experience of the problem may be the reason for their concerns. Their ideas and health beliefs may explain their expectations from the consultation, likewise their thoughts and ideas may be the reason for their preferences. This understanding is important for the doctor to avoid the usual separation of ICE (ideas, concerns and expectations) questions. The ICE are all aspects of the patient's experience of the problem and can be appreciated more fluently if the doctor is able to guide the patient through their own unique experience of the problem using reflective questions, active listening and non-verbal engagement. The questions the doctor chooses to use, especially initially in the consultation, should mostly be targeted towards encouraging and guiding the patient to 'tell their story'. It is more effective if the doctor does this with two targets in mind. First, to understand the problem enough to be able to recognise it, and secondly to develop an understanding of the patient sufficient to work in partnership with them using their shared understanding.

The doctor should know when they have achieved an understanding of the patient's experience by answering these questions during the exploration as a rough guide.

1. Why has the patient attended?

2. What do they make of the problem?

3. How would they prefer to proceed?

4. What decisions do they want to make?

5. How badly has the problem affected them?

If the doctor has these questions in mind during the data gathering, it would enhance their chances of directing the thoughts of the patient in a logical way, to encourage them to share their experience. Practising how to explore these details opportunistically, guided by the thoughts of the patient, is rewarding and improves rapport as well as the doctor's fluency and efficiency.

The dialogue below is an example of how a patient's experience is explored to develop an understanding of the patient using reflective questions, active listening and non-formulaic ICE questions.

45-year-old man

Patient: *"It's my left groin again."*

Doctor: *"Can you tell me what's happened?"*

Reflective question to show active listening to the words and meaning of what the patient has just said. The doctor recognised that the patient was describing a recurring problem, and is aware of the benefits of understanding the problem through an exploration of the patient's perspective rather than an exploration of just the problem. Questions like "Where is the pain?" would not achieve the same outcome.

> *Positive CSA indicators*
> * Explores the patient's agenda, health beliefs and preferences.
> * Appears alert to verbal and non-verbal cues.

Even at this stage the patient hasn't really given any direct information, but the doctor chooses to concentrate on gaining a description of the problem through the 'experience' of the patient. It is likely that within this context, the doctor will understand both the clinical problem and the patient.

Patient: *"You know I had pain around the scar where I had a hernia repair 5 months ago, and I rang the hospital straight away when I noticed some redness. They started me on antibiotics immediately, which resolved the problem, and I haven't had any problem with the area since then. But within the last 2 weeks, the pain has reappeared. I notice small twinges every now and then in the area when I stretch, but I haven't felt any lumps or noticed any redness or swelling. I really don't want anything to go wrong with the hernia operation."*

Patient description of the problem through their own experience of it. Doctor gains insight into the patient's reason for attending and the decision they have attended to make. However, they need to understand what the patient has made of the problem so far. The doctor now understands the patient's concerns, but it would be useful to gain an insight into the patient's understanding of the situation. This situation highlights an example of when the patient's concerns could be the reason for attending, and the patient understanding or idea could explain their concerns and expectations. These details all make up the patient's experience of the problem, and for a meaningful partnership to develop, the doctor needs to acquire this understanding early enough to be able to focus the consultation on two things: addressing the main issues that has brought the patient to them, without making any assumptions, and also keeping the patient safe using their knowledge of likelihood. Early focus on the clinical problem will distract the patient from their train of thought and discourage their continued contribution to the consultation.

> **Positive CSA indicators**
> - Explores the patient's agenda, health beliefs and preferences.
> - Appears alert to verbal and non-verbal cues.

Doctor: *"It sounds like you suspect that perhaps the same thing that happened last time is happening again."*

Reflective question aimed at developing an understanding of the patient's thoughts and expectations. The doctor demonstrates active listening, which improves rapport between the two parties because the patient feels their views are valued. This in turn makes them more likely to contribute and play a role in the consultation. This choice of question encourages the patient to share their experience. Failure to develop a grasp of the patient's understanding leads to a disjointed consultation and an inability to focus the consultation on the main tasks.

> **Negative CSA indicators**
> - Does not inquire sufficiently about the patient's perspective/health understanding.
> - Pays Insufficient attention to the patient's verbal and non-verbal communication.
> - Makes immediate assumptions about the problem.
> - Intervenes rather than using appropriate expectant management.
> - Is disorganised/unsystematic in gathering information.

Patient: *"I had a tooth infection, for which I had been taking an antibiotic for the 2 weeks before I started feeling the twinges, so I'm not sure if there's a possibility the infection may have moved from the tooth to the hernia repair. I know they put a mesh in there when they did the job, but I kept wondering if it was possible the infection may get into the mesh or something. It has really worried me."*

Patient's ideas and thoughts. These thoughts have also led to their concerns. These concerns are the underlying reason why they may have attended, and are reflected in the decision they have attended to make. It is important to understand how the patient's experience cannot be separated into different entities, as is often depicted in books. This understanding improves the doctor's fluency and efficiency when used in practice frequently.

Insufficient evidence	Needs further development	Competent	Excellent
	Develops a relationship with the patient, which works, but is focused on the problem rather than the patient.	Explores and responds to the patient's agenda, health beliefs and preferences. Elicits psychological and social information to place the patient's problem in context.	Incorporates the patient's perspective and context when negotiating the management plan.

Doctor: *"It has clearly really bothered you."*

Exploring severity and impact using opportunistic logical reflective question based on the doctor's understanding of what the patient has just said. Questions related to establishing the impact of the problem on the patient are more effective when asked in the context of the patient's own description of their experience and understanding. Questions like "How bad is it?" are very useful in understanding this context, as the context of the problem often provides the doctor with an insight into the impact of the problem, and vice versa. These are often not appreciated by candidates, who may ask a question like "How has your groin pain affected you at work?" which on its own is a closed question and may not give the doctor the scope of the impact fully.

Positive CSA indicators
- Explores the impact of the illness on the patient's life.
- Elicits psychological and social information to place the patient's problem in context.

Patient: *"I haven't done any jobs since I noticed the twinges, as I didn't want to make it any worse. I've stayed away from any strenuous activity until I can confirm for sure it isn't an infection. I don't want to have to go through another hernia surgery, as the last one left me out of a job for 2 months. My job involved a lot of lifting on the building site, so I thought I would rather miss a few days to save making it any worse. I am not in pain now but occasionally if I stretch myself I do feel a twinge. I know they said you will occasionally feel twinges after the surgery, but I was more worried about infections."*

Positive CSA indicators
- Explores the impact of the illness on the patient's life.
- Elicits psychological and social information to place the patient's problem in context.

One of the benefits of this approach to patient-centredness is that the doctor gains an early insight into the patient's experience of the problem. Putting the problem into context and providing the doctor with information related to ICE in a way that reflects a genuine interest in the patient's perspective and experience. The CSA assesses this interest and response rather than formulaic data gathering.

Positive CSA indicators
- Shows responsiveness to the patient's preferences, feelings and expectations.
- Responds to needs and concerns with interest and understanding.

The doctor uses closed questions to confirm their suspicion of scar tenderness, exclude bowel and urine problems, red flags: fevers, numbness.

This focus is achieved because the doctor recognised the problem through the narrative of the patient's experience of it. The competency recommends an ability to recognise the presentation of common problems to general practice without an exhaustive line of enquiry, and an ability to use an incremental approach to decision-making.

It is important to practise how to make decisions using probability and likelihood, at the same time maintaining the patient's safety. This can be done using selective closed questions to show the doctor's awareness of risks and uncertainties without needing to focus mainly on the clinical problem. This is a very important part of the CSA assessment and reduces significantly the length of the consultation, but in a safe manner.

Insufficient evidence	Needs further development	Competent	Excellent
From the available evidence, the doctor's performance cannot be placed on a higher point of this developmental scale.	Generates an adequate differential diagnosis based on the information available.	Makes diagnoses in a structured way using a problem-solving method. Uses an understanding of probability based on prevalence, incidence and natural history of illness to aid decision-making. Addresses problems that present early and/or in an undifferentiated way by integrating all the available information to help generate a differential diagnosis. Uses time as a diagnostic tool.	Uses pattern recognition to identify diagnoses quickly, safely and reliably. Remains aware of the limitations of pattern recognition and when to revert to an analytical approach.

Doctor: *"Is it OK for me to have a look at the area to help me clarify what might be going on?"*

Examination: no recurrence. Healthy wound. No tenderness. Temp NAD.

Focused examination enough to clarify the suspicion and allay the patient's concerns. The examination should demonstrate a logical attempt for the doctor to clarify the likely diagnosis or in some cases exclude unlikely causes.

Doctor: *"I can't find any evidence of an infection in the scar from your previous surgery. Although I understand your thoughts about the infection you had in the tooth, there isn't any way the infection could have gone into the scar. I think you're right about the twinges that can* *happen from time to time within the area where the hernia was repaired, especially when stretched, but that doesn't necessarily mean an infection. The scar would have been red if it had become infected, just like you noticed the previous time. I think you should be able to continue working as the area of the wound should have healed quite well by now."*

Explanations can be medically correct but still not regarded as enhanced enough to improve the patient's understanding. Any explanation not only needs to be understandable, it also needs to be relevant to the patient. A doctor who explores ICE, for instance, without genuinely acquiring that information with an intention to empower the patient, is less likely to respond to that understanding when giving the patient information.

> *Positive CSA indicators*
> - Shows responsiveness to the patient's preferences, feelings and expectations.
> - Provides explanations that are relevant and understandable to the patient.

The doctor has also explored and responded to the patient's perspective by offering an explanation which reflects that understanding.

Insufficient evidence	Needs further development	Competent	Excellent
From the available evidence, the doctor's performance cannot be placed on a higher point of this developmental scale.	Provides explanations that are medically correct but doctor-centred.	Uses the patient's understanding to help improve the explanation offered.	Uses a variety of communication techniques and materials (e.g. written or electronic) to adapt explanations to the needs of the patient.

The doctor uses his understanding of the patient's views to improve the explanation he has offered to the patient. This is one of the opportunities presented in the CSA for the doctor to demonstrate their understanding of patient-centredness. An explanation like "I've examined your groin, and the wound looks all OK" will not achieve the task, and will fail to demonstrate good interpersonal skills. The patient's agenda remains unresolved, and although the explanation is medically correct, the patient's reason for attending remains unaddressed, as the explanation may not have allayed their worst fears.

From the above, it is clear that in some cases the content of the patient's side of the story and experience may enhance the doctor's understanding of the reason for the patient's attendance. If, however, this is assumed from the start without clarification, this may result in a poorly structured consultation which is unable to achieve the task of the consultation, despite a thorough, conventional history taking. Even if that is partially achieved, it may be unlikely to achieve the task in response to the preference of the patient in a timely manner.

Insufficient evidence	Needs further development	Competent	Excellent
	Uses a rigid or formulaic approach to achieve the main tasks of the consultation.	Achieves the tasks of the consultation, responding to the preferences of the patient in an efficient manner.	Appropriately uses advanced consultation skills, such as confrontation or catharsis, to achieve better patient outcomes.

Chapter 7

Managing uncertainty, sharing risks

One of the unique features of patient-centredness and focused consultations is the ability it gives the doctor to manage problems at an early undifferentiated stage, and to share the risk of those uncertainties with the patient when necessary. The doctor is expected to communicate the risk effectively to the patient, and involve the patient in its management to the appropriate degree.[1] To achieve this, the doctor recognises the uncertainty, especially where it is related to the patient's concerns, and gathers enough information to understand the nature of the clinical condition and the patient's experience of it, but demonstrates their ability to tolerate these uncertainties using their knowledge of likelihoods and good clinical knowledge of the natural course of common conditions. With the understanding of the patient, the doctor is able to take their patient's views into account in the decision-making so that the thoughts and feelings of both parties are considered during the planning of management of the uncertainty, thereby empowering the patient and enhancing the patient's autonomy. When the consultation is approached in this way, patients understand the basis of the doctor's thought process, improving their compliance with the agreed course of action. The doctor uses red flags and targeted safety nets to show their understanding of the course of illnesses and uncertainties, to keep the consultation safe.

> *Positive CSA indicator*
> - Uses an incremental approach, using time and accepting uncertainty.

Insufficient evidence	Needs further development	Competent	Excellent
	Identifies and tolerates uncertainties in the consultation, but struggles to reassure the patient or to manage them independently.	Is able to manage uncertainty, including that experienced by the patient.	Anticipates and employs a variety of strategies for managing uncertainty.

The case below is a dialogue involving the sharing of risk, demonstrating how partnership and rapport can enhance the process.

58-year-old woman on perindopril 8 mg (BP 114/70 last week)

Patient: *"I haven't felt right for the last few months, doctor."*

Patient's opening statement is vague. Although the doctor recognises the value of allowing the patient to tell their story and share their thoughts and experiences, it is important to be flexible with the order of the approach. In this case the doctor needs to clarify the nature of the problem first, but this is done more effectively by using a line of enquiry that is likely to encourage the patient to give a description of the symptoms using their experience of the problem. It is likely that within that context, the doctor may gain some insight into the nature of the decision the patient has attended to make, their thoughts about the problem and their reason for attending. These often require the doctor to pay careful attention and listen actively to what the patient is describing: reflective questions are more exploratory and rewarding when they are used as an enquiry to reflect back to the patient, using paraphrases to confirm to the patient that they have been heard.

Doctor: *"What's been happening?"*

Reflective question to explore both the problem and the patient's experience of it. The doctor demonstrates an awareness of the benefit of using selective questions, which improves the doctor's insight into the patient's experience of the problem, without focusing on just the problem. The nature of the problem is recognised through its description by the patient.

> *Positive CSA indicators*
> - Gathers information from history taking, examination and investigation in a systematic and efficient manner.
> - Is appropriately selective in the choice of enquiries, examinations and investigations.

Patient: *"I saw one of your colleagues last week regarding how I was feeling. He arranged a few blood tests as we talked about perhaps excluding anaemia or other causes, but I gather the blood tests have all come back OK. We couldn't work out what would be the cause of the head rush I was experiencing. The other day I felt lightheaded after having a meal at the restaurant, and needed a drink of water to gather myself. It happened just as I got up to go to the bathroom, but I recovered quite quickly and I didn't need to call an ambulance. I have felt well since then, although this last occasion was the third time it's happened within the last 6 months. I can't just carry on like this without doing anything about it."*

The doctor is able to appreciate the frustration expressed by the patient about the ongoing problem and the lack of diagnosis. There are cues here for the doctor to develop more insight into the impact of the situation and put the problems into context. It is beneficial to avoid interrupting the train of thought of the patient, and continue to encourage their contribution. This not only improves the patient's participation, but enhances rapport and partnership. The history of the clinical problem can also be sought first, as long as the doctor is aware that they will need to keep the consultation open at this stage, following a logical line of questioning focused on discovering the patient's reason for attending. Within this context, the doctor should develop an understanding of the clinical problem presentation through recognition of its features using likelihood. This early recognition of the pattern of the condition improves the doctor's efficiency by using closed questions to clarify the likely cause, excluding red flags.

> *Positive CSA indicators*
> - Clarifies the problem and nature of decision required.
> - Uses an incremental approach, using time and accepting uncertainty.
> - Gathers information from history taking, examination and investigation in a systematic and efficient manner.

Doctor: *"It sounds like it has bothered you quite a bit."*

Empathy. Reflective question to gain understanding into the severity and effect on the patient. Gives the doctor an understanding of the problem in context. This understanding will influence the doctor's explanation and management approaches. The doctor recognises that this question is likely to give the patient an opportunity to share their inner thoughts and concerns.

Questions like "How bad has it been?" are likely to achieve a similar outcome, but a question which focuses on the clinical problem at this stage is likely to distract the patient from their train of thought and may impair their contributions.

Patient: *"It has made me very anxious about going out because I don't know when and where it will occur. It's difficult to cope with a problem if you don't understand what's causing it, or what one might be doing to bring it on. I have checked all the things I've done recently to see whether there may be any connections or anything causing it. I run a shop which involves standing for long periods, and I get very worried about fainting in front of my customers, which is why I was hoping that the blood test would show something wrong."*

Impact of the problem. Psychological and physical. Patient's understanding. This information gives the doctor an ability to put the problem into context, to empathise more appropriately, and to respond or achieve any task in this consultation in partnership.

Insufficient evidence	Needs further development	Competent	Excellent
From the available evidence, the doctor's performance cannot be placed on a higher point of this developmental scale.	Recognises the impact of the problem on the patient.	Recognises the impact of the problem on the patient, their family and/or carers.	Recognises and shows understanding of the limits of the doctor's ability to intervene in the holistic care of the patient.

Positive CSA indicators
- Explores the impact of the illness on the patient's life.
- Elicits psychological and social information to place the patient's problem in context.

Doctor: *"What kind of shop is it?"*

Opportunistic social context. Logical structure.

Questions asked in the CSA that are out of context are considered as non-systematic and a poorly structured approach and are a negative indicator. This is a common cause of failure and often a result of poor understanding of the competency framework.

The impact of a problem often puts the problem in the context of its experience by the patient.

Negative CSA indicators
- Is disorganised/unsystematic in gathering information.
- Data gathering does not appear to be guided by the probabilities of disease.

Patient: *"I sell hair products."*

Doctor: *"From what you have said, it sounds like you've been thinking about the causes."*

Non-formulaic way of seeking patient's understanding using a reflective paraphrase to reassure the patient that their views are being heard and taken seriously, encouraging further contributions.

> *Positive CSA indicators*
> - Explores patient's agenda, health beliefs and preferences.
> - Appears alert to verbal and non-verbal cues.

Patient: *"I wasn't sure whether I was taking something I may be allergic to, although I only take perindopril and no other medications and I've been on the tablets for my BP for over 10 years without any problems."*

Patient's understanding and thoughts. The value of the patient's views is seen in the decision-making stages, as the doctor is able to work in partnership with the patient. They can only find a common ground if they have developed an understanding of the patient's views, especially when the diagnosis may be undifferentiated or uncertain. It is much easier to communicate risk to a patient if the doctor understands the patient's views.

> *Positive CSA indicators*
> - Works in partnership, finding common ground to develop a shared management plan.
> - Communicates risk effectively to patients.

Signposting. Doctor clarifies the postural nature of the symptoms using closed questions, but this should be done in a way that shows their understanding of the natural courses of the common causes. The doctor recognises the likely cause from the description, but uses their knowledge of possible alternatives to choose appropriate selective question to exclude red flags. Using their understanding of the patient's views, the doctor also clarifies the timing of the dose of the medication and previous blood pressures taken by the patient. The doctor excludes red flags: chest pains, palpitations, neurological symptoms during episodes, headaches, weight changes. Drug compliance. Allergies.

The ability to use the understanding of the patient to recognise the likely cause and focus the data gathering to achieve a confirmation of possible causes of the problem, after excluding red flags, is an important skill to develop, as it improves the doctor's efficiency. This requires a good knowledge of the use of safety nets and patient involvement. An excellent candidate is able to identify the scope of enquiry needed to explore the problem within a very short time frame, and this is developed through regular practice day to day, but using the right understanding of the competency.

> *Positive CSA indicator*
> - Is appropriately selective in the choice of enquiries, examinations and investigations.

Insufficient evidence	Needs further development	Competent	Excellent
	Accumulates information from the patient that is mainly relevant to their problem. Uses existing information in the patient records.	Systematically gathers information, using questions appropriately targeted to the problem without affecting patient safety. Understands the importance of, and makes appropriate use of, existing information about the problem and the patient's context.	Expertly identifies the nature and scope of enquiry needed to investigate the problem, or multiple problems, within a short time-frame. Prioritises problems in a way that enhances patient satisfaction.

Doctor: *"I think it would help me if I could measure your blood pressure and examine your heart. Is that OK?"*

Examination: no pallor, pulse 80 regular. BP 114/72 mmHg, no postural changes, normal CVS. Normal central and peripheral neurology.

No causes found. Normal routine blood screen.

Doctor: *"You're right that all the tests have come back OK, and there's nothing to show that you are anaemic. From the description of the head rush, it sounds like the problem happens more often when you stand after sitting or lying for a while. This may suggest perhaps a change in your blood pressure occasionally when you change position. I was wondering, as you mentioned, whether the tablets may have something to do with it. I know you've been on them for a few years, but occasionally the blood pressure may become a little lower with time than it was originally when you started taking the tablets years ago. The reading today is normal but a little on the low side. It doesn't mean you have become allergic to the tablets, but it may be that the dose you're taking may be a little too high for you. There are no signs to suggest that anything else more sinister might be causing the dizziness, from your examination."*

The explanation demonstrates a response by the doctor to their understanding of the patient, offering information in a way to make it relevant to the patient's experience and thoughts. The doctor uses suggestions in offering their thoughts and opinions, but explaining those thoughts. The use of information elicited from the patient, when offering them an explanation is a useful way to continue to encourage the patient's participation in the partnership.

Insufficient evidence	Needs further development	Competent	Excellent
From the available evidence, the doctor's performance cannot be placed on a higher point of this developmental scale.	Provides explanations that are medically correct but doctor-centred.	Uses the patient's understanding to help improve the explanation offered.	Uses a variety of communication techniques and materials (e.g. written or electronic) to adapt explanations to the needs of the patient.

> *Positive CSA indicators*
> - Provides explanations that are relevant and understandable to the patient.
> - Shows responsiveness to the patient's preferences, feelings and expectations.
> - Enhances patient autonomy.

Patient: *"That would make sense, because it does happen more often towards midday, a few hours after taking the tablet."*

Giving the patient an opportunity to get involved in decision-making.

> *Positive CSA indicators*
> - Works in partnership, finding common ground to develop a shared management plan.
> - Communicates risk effectively to patients.
> - Shows responsiveness to the patient's preferences, feelings and expectations.
> - Enhances patient autonomy.

Doctor: *"One way we can be sure of the cause of the problem would be to reduce the amount of medication you're taking, to see if it resolves the problem. Perhaps taking only half of your normal amount for a period of 2 weeks."*

Offering patient suggestions gives them an opportunity to be involved in the decision-making, especially when they understand the explanation offered by the doctor. The doctor uses their understanding of the natural history of common conditions in offering options. The ability to offer a tailored option that is relevant and feasible to the patient is more effective when done on the basis that the patient feels empowered and part of the decision-making, thereby enhancing autonomy.

Insufficient evidence	Needs further development	Competent	Excellent
	Makes decisions by applying rules, plans or protocols.	Thinks flexibly around problems, generating functional solutions.	No longer relies on rules or protocols but is able to use and justify discretionary judgement in situations of uncertainty or complexity, for example in patients with multiple problems.

> *Positive CSA indicators*
> - Makes plans that reflect the natural history of common problems.
> - Offers appropriate and feasible management options.

Patient: *"What if my blood pressure goes up?"*

Working in partnership, patient empowered to participate in decision-making. This participation is the only way to achieve a mutually agreed plan, and the negotiation is only significant if done on the basis that the parties involved have been able to share with each other their thoughts and feelings about the situation.

Insufficient evidence	Needs further development	Competent	Excellent
	Communicates management plans but without negotiating with, or involving, the patient.	Works in partnership with the patient, negotiating a mutually acceptable plan that respects the patient's agenda and preference for involvement.	Whenever possible, adopts plans that respect the patient's autonomy. When there is a difference of opinion the patient's autonomy is respected and a positive relationship is maintained.

Doctor: *"The blood pressure reading is very good today, and I wouldn't expect it to creep up to a dangerous level if we cut the dose to half. We could monitor the blood pressure readings to make sure it doesn't change significantly within that time frame."*

Using an understanding of the natural course of a condition to aid decision-making. Decision-making is expected to show the doctor's understanding of risks and problem solving. They should be able to weigh up the options using their knowledge of risk to guide the patient with the decision-making, and not make the decisions for the patient.

Insufficient evidence	Needs further development	Competent	Excellent
	Generates an adequate differential diagnosis based on the information available.	Makes diagnoses in a structured way using a problem-solving method. Uses an understanding of probability based on prevalence, incidence and natural history of illness to aid decision-making.	Uses pattern recognition to identify diagnoses quickly, safely and reliably. Remains aware of the limitations of pattern recognition and when to revert to an analytical approach.

Negative CSA indicators
- Instructs the patient rather than seeking common ground.
- Uses a rigid approach to consulting that fails to be sufficiently responsive to the patient's contribution.
- Fails to empower the patient or encourage self-sufficiency.

Doctor: *"I would recommend that we meet again within 2 weeks to see how you feel on the lower dose and also to check your blood pressure and make sure it has remained OK. I would expect the symptoms you were getting to ease or resolve if we are right about the decision, but if within that time, you notice any new symptoms like headache, changes in your vision or the episodes happening even more, you must let me know. If you experience any problems when the surgery is closed, you will need to use the 'out of hours' number to seek medical advice."*

Safety net, taking into account the uncertainties of the consultation. The CSA assesses how the doctor uses safety nets to demonstrate the inherent uncertainties experienced by doctors who consult in a focused patient-centred way within a limited time. The doctor should understand the value of using a safety net that reflects the decision they have made with the patient during the negotiations and the risks of the uncertainties of the presentation. A safety net which is offered in a formulaic manner without taking the uncertainties of the consultation into account is considered as disjointed and ineffective, for example "If not better, come back".

Positive CSA indicators
- Manages risk effectively, safety netting appropriately.
- Makes plans that reflect the natural history of common problems.

Chapter 8

How to use the patient's perspective to find a practical solution

Sometimes doctors approach the CSA with some apprehension that they may encounter a case where they don't know the full details of the management of the condition that the patient has attended to address.[2] Knowledge of the management of common conditions is important for dealing with the patient's problem, but a patient-centred approach provides a unique opportunity for the doctor to use their broad knowledge and experience to find practical and functional solutions to the patient's problem using problem solving. Functional solutions are achieved by the doctor thinking flexibly around problems, using their understanding of the patient's unique experience of the problem. In other words, the CSA expects the doctor to have a good knowledge of the management of common conditions, but what is assessed is the use of that knowledge to manage the condition as it applies to that individual patient's experience. This tailoring or varying of the management plan is achieved by learning how to efficiently develop an understanding of the patient. The use of rigid rules and protocols in managing the patient's problems is a negative indicator, especially if the doctor does not show responsiveness to their understanding of the patient's unique experience.

Insufficient evidence	Needs further development	Competent	Excellent
	Uses appropriate but limited management options without taking into account the preferences of the patient. Makes decisions by applying rules, plans or protocols.	Varies management options responsively according to the circumstances, priorities and preferences of those involved. Thinks flexibly around problems, generating functional solutions.	Provides patient-centred management plans whilst taking account of local and national guidelines in a timely manner. No longer relies on rules or protocols but is able to use and justify discretionary judgement in situations of uncertainty or complexity, for example in patients with multiple problems.

Positive CSA indicators
- Offers appropriate and feasible management options.
- Shows responsiveness to the patient's preferences, feelings and expectations.

The dialogue below shows a typical CSA case to demonstrate how functional solutions can be achieved by working in partnership with the patient, using patient-centredness.

14-year-old girl attending with her mother

Patient's mother: *"She can't just sleep again doctor. I wanted to have a chat with you because she seems to have developed anxiety towards everything. She has asked me to do a lot of the talking for her, and I hope that would be ok."*

Opening statement. The doctor considers the line of thought of the patient using active listening to determine the best way to encourage the patient to share their inner thoughts of the situation, to gain insight into the real reason for the patient's attendance. The choice of question the doctor chooses at this stage should be aimed at developing that insight. Generic questions like "Tell me more" may not indicate good active listening, as it would appear the doctor didn't hear or understand what the patient has just said. A good way to develop an understanding of the patient's experience of the problem is to learn how to make enquiries that allow the patient to share their thoughts and feelings without any interruptions. This can sometimes be achieved by just a non-verbal gesture from the doctor or even silence, but the most effective, from practice, is the use of a selective reflective question aimed at encouraging the patient's contributions, so that the problem presented can be put into the context of the patient's experience. It is within this context that the doctor should be able to understand and clarify the nature of the decision the patient has attended to make or clarify the main task to achieve the level of focus required to conduct the rest of the consultation fluently and efficiently.

Positive CSA indicator
- Clarifies the problem and nature of decision required.

Negative CSA indicator
- Makes immediate assumptions about the problem.

Doctor: *"Can you tell me what's been happening?"*

Reflective question demonstrating the doctor's understanding of the ongoing nature of her problem from her comments, encouraging the patient to share the story of the event leading up to their attendance. This question is aimed at allowing the patient to describe the problem in the context of their experience of it, and the doctor may gain an insight into the reason for the patient's attendance while at the same time recognising the condition the patient has presented with. Doctors who approach the consultation in this way are likely to gain an insight to allow them to focus the rest of the consultation. The doctor's focus at this point is mainly on accumulating information from the patient that is mainly relevant to their experience of it rather than just to the clinical problem.

Insufficient evidence	Needs further development	Competent	Excellent
	Accumulates information from the patient that is mainly relevant to their problem. Uses existing information in the patient records.	Systematically gathers information, using questions appropriately targeted to the problem without affecting patient safety. Understands the importance of, and makes appropriate use of, existing information about the problem and the patient's context.	Expertly identifies the nature and scope of enquiry needed to investigate the problem, or multiple problems, within a short time-frame. Prioritises problems in a way that enhances patient satisfaction.

The details of the patient's experience of the problem are likely to put the problem in context, and provide an opportunity for the doctor to understand the impact of the problem on the patient and others. It is important to learn how to use the description of the problem by the patient to pick out opportunities to explore sufficiently the patient's perspective of the problem. In some consultations, the doctor needs to understand that they can be flexible as to choice of line of initial enquiry to adapt to the style of the patient or the nature of the complaint, as they may occasionally need to explore the problem first to recognise the clinical condition and also gain some insight into the patient's experience of the problem.

Insufficient evidence	Needs further development	Competent	Excellent
	Demonstrates a limited range of data gathering styles and methods.	Demonstrates different styles of data gathering and adapts these to a wide range of patients and situations.	Able to gather information in a wide range of circumstances and across all patient groups (including their family and representatives) in a sensitive, empathetic and ethical manner.

Patient's mother: *"She had several counselling sessions in school last year for her feelings after she was bullied. The school has sorted all that out now, but recently she seems to have become a little more anxious than normal. The main problem is that she's struggling to get to sleep, staying awake sometimes till midnight in her room. She's in year 10 now, and I'm not sure whether all the pressures from school for GCSEs might be affecting her. I wasn't sure whether there is anything that can be done."*

Patient's mother shares the story and within this story the doctor should recognise the line of thoughts of the patient. The doctor needs to clarify the exact nature of the problem, the exact reason for this attendance, and the nature of the decision the patient has attended to make. This insight is gained from encouraging the patient's contribution in the consultation, and in this case the doctor explores the problem but from the perspective of the patient's experience. The doctor uses reflective questions to explore the nature of the experience of the problem by the patient so they can gain an overall holistic view of the problem in context. Developing the understanding of the problem in this context provides an opportunity for the doctor to empathise more appropriately. It also enhances rapport, improves insight into the patient's reason for attending and focuses the consultation.

Insufficient evidence	Needs further development	Competent	Excellent
From the available evidence, the doctor's performance cannot be placed on a higher point of this developmental scale.	Recognises the impact of the problem on the patient.	Recognises the impact of the problem on the patient, their family and/or carers.	Recognises and shows understanding of the limits of the doctor's ability to intervene in the holistic care of the patient.

Positive CSA indicators
- Explores the impact of the illness on the patient's life.
- Elicits psychological and social information to place the patient's problem in context.

Doctor: *"It sounds like it has been difficult. Can you describe what happens in a typical night?"*

Empathy. The doctor understands the problem by using an open description from the patient's experience by using a reflective question to encourage more contribution from the patient's perspective of the situation. Focusing on the problem at this stage may not explore the patient's experience sufficiently to reveal the exact nature of the reason for attending, and the doctor may not be able to clarify fully the nature of the decision needing to be made.

Positive CSA indicators
- Clarifies the problem and nature of decision required.
- Gathers information efficiently, taking into account the uniqueness of the patient.
- Is selective in the choice of the enquiries and examination.

The doctor can only be selective in their choice of enquiry from this point if they are able to clarify the tasks the patient has attended to deal with, and developed an understanding of the patient's point of view. Otherwise, they are likely to be too broad and inefficient with their enquiry, requiring longer consultation times.

Negative CSA indicators
- Is disorganised/unsystematic in gathering information.
- Data gathering does not appear to be guided by the probabilities of disease.

Patient: *"I go to bed only when mum tells me to do so, usually around 10pm or so. I normally spend some time on my phone to keep my mind occupied until probably around 11pm, but when I try to sleep my mind will be occupied with thoughts of school and all the work. Some days I've gone into my sister's room if I can't get off to sleep, as she makes me feel comfortable by talking to me. I don't like going into her room really, as it feels like I'm invading her space. I eventually get off to sleep, usually a few minutes after midnight."*

The doctor understands the impact of the problem on others. The impact of a problem, the patient's concerns and their expectation are all potential reasons for the patient's attendance, and should not be seen as simply a routine enquiry in history taking, as they often determine the tasks of the consultation as seen from the patient's point of view. For example, a patient attends with a complaint of feeling 'shaky', and the doctor proceeds to verify from the patient their experience of the problem in an open manner. He discovers they have been trying to get themselves off a painkiller they have been taking for a few months. On exploring this further, the doctor discovers that the patient decided to come off these tablets because their wedding was coming up in 2 weeks' time, and they had read on a leaflet that they are unable to have a glass of wine whilst on the tablet. This depth of context and understanding of the patient's experience focuses the rest of the consultation to deal with the task that the patient has presented with. An inability to explore the patient's understanding in this way is likely to result in an inefficient consultation. Establishing this context early is a very important part of the CSA assessment.

Negative CSA indicator
- Does not appreciate the impact of the patient's psychosocial context.

Insufficient evidence	Needs further development	Competent	Excellent
	Enquires into physical, psychological and social aspects of the patient's problem.	Demonstrates understanding of the patient in relation to their socio-economic and cultural background. The doctor uses this understanding to inform discussion and to generate practical suggestions for the management of the patient.	Accesses information about the patient's psycho-social history in a fluent and non-judgemental manner that puts the patient at ease.

Doctor: *"How has it been at school?"*

Verbal cue. Gaining understanding of the patient's experience of the problem. Putting the problem into a social context. At this stage the doctor is using their understanding of the common reasons for a 14-year-old to have sleep problems, to discover the most likely cause of the problem. Doctors struggle with thoughts of getting the right diagnosis, but the competency assessed is the ability of the doctor to use an understanding of probability based on prevalence, and natural history of the illness to aid decision-making. It's uncommon in general practice to be precise about the definitive diagnosis, as conditions do not always present as a typical textbook description, but an understanding of the use of likelihood and problem solving guided by the doctor's knowledge of the natural course of a condition is more important, and strong knowledge of red flags reflected in the strength of the safety net offered.

Patient's mother: *"School has been fine. She does all her homework, but I suspect she may be under a little bit of pressure as she doesn't pick up things in school as well as her sisters. She is well supported at home, and we all help out with her homework when we can. Her grades are reasonable. There haven't been any problems reported from school recently, but she has never really liked school."*

Context. The patient's description can sometimes reassure the doctor of the direction of focus, as the mother is clearly indicating that the school performances are OK. It appears that the pressures from school work might be an issue.

Positive CSA indicator
- Data gathering appears to be guided by the probabilities of disease.

Doctor: *"Have you had any chats with the school regarding the current struggles?"*

The doctor gains an insight into the most likely cause of her problem. Preparing a common ground for discussion later in the consultation using this understanding. Explores the thoughts of the patient's mother regarding possible interventions. Finding a practical solution to assist the patient, discovering patient's preference. Often questions like "Have you had this before?", or "What helped previously?" are useful in understanding the patient's thoughts about an intervention, and their preferences.

> *Positive CSA indicator*
> * Offers appropriate and feasible management options.

Patient's mother: *"I've discussed this with Charlotte, but she did say she wouldn't want to have counselling in school like she had last year. She feels shy about what her friends would say if she attends counselling at school. She actually benefited from the support last year, but I was reluctant to approach the school because of how she felt. I wasn't sure whether there is any counselling she could have in the community to help her get through this difficulty."*

Patient's concerns and preferences discovered through active listening, encouraging the patient to share their views in partnership with the doctor. Exploring data required for decision-making is usually only possible if the doctor is able to foresee those possibilities and negotiations early using their knowledge of the management of common presentations – this is a skill expected in the CSA.

> *Positive CSA indicator*
> * Recognises presentations of common physical, psychological and social problems.

Doctor uses closed questions to clarify how she feels during other times in the day, and at weekends. Clarifies whether any other features of concern. Clarifies systemic health. Excludes red flags, i.e. thoughts of harm.

This focus is achieved because of the doctor's understanding of the problem, forming a view of the most likely cause of the problem. The doctor keeps the patient safe using closed questions to complete their agenda. Often doctors approach the CSA by spending the majority of the time focusing on the problem rather the patient's experience of the problem, failing to discover the reason for attending and the main task through developing an understanding of the problem in the patient's context. This is a common cause of failure in the CSA examination.

> *Positive CSA indicators*
> * Gathers information from history taking, examination and investigation in a systematic and efficient manner.
> * Is appropriately selective in the choice of enquiries, examinations and investigations.

Doctor: *"It sounds like the major cause of Charlotte's poor sleep is more linked to the situation at school, especially as she feels much better over the weekends and on holidays. I know you were considering some support in the community for her, especially now that the pressures of GCSEs are piling up."*

The doctor shares their own thoughts but is offering an explanation using a language which reflects their understanding of the patient's experience.

Insufficient evidence	Needs further development	Competent	Excellent
From the available evidence, the doctor's performance cannot be placed on a higher point of this developmental scale.	Provides explanations that are medically correct but doctor-centred.	Uses the patient's understanding to help improve the explanation offered.	Uses a variety of communication techniques and materials (e.g. written or electronic) to adapt explanations to the needs of the patient.

It's important to note that explanations that are medically correct or non-jargon can still be doctor-centred, if the doctor does not respond to their understanding of the patient's experience. The explanation has to demonstrate a realistic benefit of gathering information from the patient's perspective. Doctors in the CSA sometimes gather information related to the patient's perspective without using this understanding to improve the explanation they offer to the patient. This is a negative indicator in the CSA. The competency requires doctors to '**explore**' and '**respond**' to the patient's perspective, as this is part of the benefit of working in partnership with the patient.

Insufficient evidence	Needs further development	Competent	Excellent
	Develops a relationship with the patient, which works, but is focused on the problem rather than the patient.	Explores and responds to the patient's agenda, health beliefs and preferences. Elicits psychological and social information to place the patient's problem in context.	Incorporates the patient's perspective and context when negotiating the management plan.

Doctor: *"I understand Charlotte's difficulties with school-based counselling, and I agree it sounds like there would be a benefit from support. There are services in the community that can support her through the difficulties at school, but I'm not sure whether they would be able to provide her with the level of support she might receive from the counselling in school. Normally the school counsellor will have more idea of the goings-on with her studies and those pressures, and perhaps provide the best direct support for her progress. They may be able to monitor her progress better. Services in the community can often involve a bit of a wait to get seen, and I'm not sure if perhaps she needs some support that can be put in place sooner than later. I'm not sure how you feel about that."*

Doctor offers an option, responding to their understanding of the patient's concerns and preferences. The management is offered in an incremental manner, taking into account the patient's experience of the problem. The doctor tailors the management to the patient's situation. Statements like "I will refer you for counselling" made in a generic way should be avoided in the CSA. The doctor should always consider suggesting options that are feasible and appropriate for the patient's unique situation and context, showing their responsiveness. The best way to achieve this task is by working in partnership with the patient, pre-empting the discussions to gain an understanding of the nature of the decision the patient has attended to make, finding a common ground by understanding how the patient feels about the option beforehand through developing an understanding of the patient's thoughts and preferences. For example, it would be a negative indicator to offer a patient an option of using a suppository for constipation if they have already tried using suppositories for many years without any effect. The doctor should have recognised the possible interventions that may be indicated and pre-empted that negotiation by establishing the patient's views beforehand to enable them to tailor their advice.

Insufficient evidence	Needs further development	Competent	Excellent
	Uses a rigid or formulaic approach to achieve the main tasks of the consultation.	Achieves the tasks of the consultation, responding to the preferences of the patient in an efficient manner.	Appropriately uses advanced consultation skills, such as confrontation or catharsis, to achieve better patient outcomes.

Patient's mother: *"I can see what you mean. I thought about the wait actually. I may have to speak to the counsellor myself, and also share Charlotte's concerns with her to see if they can suggest any ways around the problem."*

Mutual agreement. The patient feels empowered to accept the decision based on their understanding of the thoughts of the doctor.

Doctor: *"We can always review the decision and try a different option if there are difficulties. In the meantime, we may have to think about agreeing on a bedtime routine."*

Safety net.

> **Positive CSA indicator**
> - Manages risk effectively, safety netting appropriately.

Patient's mother: *"We had the conversation yesterday, and we agreed on a bedtime of 9.30 pm. I've also talked to her about using the phone after bedtime as that keeps your head going, doesn't it?"*

Health promotion.

> **Positive CSA indicators**
> - Encourages improvement, rehabilitation and, where appropriate, recovery.
> - Encourages the patient to participate in appropriate health promotion and disease prevention strategies.

Chapter 9

Data gathering to develop understanding of the problem and the patient simultaneously

The CSA assesses the doctor's fluency in their ability to recognise the nature of the clinical problem presented by the patient, and also to develop an understanding of the patient's perspective.[1] The examination then assesses how the doctor demonstrates responsiveness to the acquired understanding of the patient. The data gathering domain focuses on the understanding of the patient's problem through the patient's perspective, the clinical management domain assesses how decisions are made in partnership with the patient and the interpersonal skill domain assesses how the doctor demonstrates responsiveness to their understanding of the patient's perspective. The importance of sufficiently exploring the patient's perspective in any encounter – regardless of the nature of the clinical problem presented – is shown in the connection between the three domains of assessment of the CSA.

1. The data gathering domain assesses how the doctor focuses this data gathering using their understanding of the reasons for the patient's attendance. This means choosing the line of enquiry, which is guided by the probability and likelihood, and focusing on the decisions the patient has attended to make.

2. The clinical management domain assesses how the doctor uses his knowledge of the patient and the problem to tailor the management options offered. This means being aware of the patient's experience of the problem and their context, to find a common ground with the patient.

3. The interpersonal skill domain assesses how the doctor explores and responds to the uniqueness of the patient through building rapport, genuine empathy, and involving the patient throughout the consultation.

These three aspects are clearly all linked to patient-centredness and should not be seen as separate entities. A common misunderstanding is to assume a doctor may do well in clinical management even when they haven't shown good interpersonal skills, as it is clear the three domains are centred around the patient rather than the problem presented by the patient.

47-year-old man

Patient: *"I've experienced this pain around my elbows over the last 2 weeks. I'm not really sure what's caused it, but it feels to me it might be deep in the bones. I don't feel any pains on the bone itself when I press on the area, but the pain is right on the outside part of the* *elbow. I can't remember hurting the area at all so I was wondering if you could have a look and tell me what it could be."*

Understanding of the patient's reason for attending can be gained more effectively by encouraging the patient to share their thoughts and feelings of the problem freely without interruption. A fluent practitioner will learn how to recognise the nature of the common condition presented within the context of the simultaneous exploration of the patient's views. If the doctor is unable to clarify the task of the consultation at this stage, it might be difficult for them to focus the rest of the data gathering to the particular issues that are important to the patient, and may focus mainly on the doctor's agenda. The main objective of the consultation is for the doctor to diagnose the problem the patient has presented with, and manage that problem in such a way that they involve the patient in the decision-making. It is clear that without sufficiently understanding the patient's point of view or preferences, this process will become very difficult to accomplish. Although the patient has attended with a pain in the elbow, for instance, the doctor needs to know what the problem means to the patient, how they would like to be treated, what they have already tried previously, etc. to then be able to look at finding a common ground for negotiations.

> *Positive CSA indicator*
> - Clarifies the problem and nature of decision required.

Insufficient evidence	Needs further development	Competent	Excellent
	Accumulates information from the patient that is mainly relevant to their problem. Uses existing information in the patient records.	Systematically gathers information, using questions appropriately targeted to the problem without affecting patient safety. Understands the importance of, and makes appropriate use of, existing information about the problem and the patient's context.	Expertly identifies the nature and scope of enquiry needed to investigate the problem, or multiple problems, within a short time-frame. Prioritises problems in a way that enhances patient satisfaction.

Doctor: *"When you said it feels like it's in the bone, what did you mean exactly?"*

Verbal cues. Reflective questioning demonstrating active listening. The doctor explores the patient's understanding and interpretation of the problem. Patients share their unique experience of a problem when they perceive the doctor's willingness to understand that experience. This understanding is likely to place the patient's complaint into the right context, and may improve the doctor's insight into the exact reason for attending.

> *Positive CSA indicators*
> - Clarifies the problem and nature of decision required.
> - Explores the patient's agenda, health beliefs and preferences.
> - Appears alert to verbal and non-verbal cues.

Patient: *"I can't really remember hurting that part of my elbow, and I couldn't work out any particular reason the pain would have started. The pain feels very deep inside. My father passed away 2 years ago after battling unsuccessfully with a very nasty lymphoma and he didn't seek any medical attention early when he was having aches and pains. I remember the doctor mentioning at the time that his cancer may have spread in the bones so since I started feeling this pain, I have looked up on the lymphoma website but really I haven't got any of the other signs mentioned there for lymphoma as I feel so well in myself. I thought perhaps my new blood pressure tablets might be causing the pain as it does say on the leaflet about muscle pains, but the pain hasn't really changed since I stopped them. I really don't know what to make of it at all."*

Doctor gains an understanding of the reason for patient's attendance. Empathises more appropriately using this understanding, understands the patient's concerns and thoughts. This was possible because the doctor used a reflective question to explore and develop a relationship with the patient rather than focusing on obtaining a history of the elbow pain.

Insufficient evidence	Needs further development	Competent	Excellent
	Accumulates information from the patient that is mainly relevant to their problem. Uses existing information in the patient records.	Systematically gathers information, using questions appropriately targeted to the problem without affecting patient safety. Understands the importance of, and makes appropriate use of, existing information about the problem and the patient's context.	Expertly identifies the nature and scope of enquiry needed to investigate the problem, or multiple problems, within a short time-frame. Prioritises problems in a way that enhances patient satisfaction.

Doctor: *"I'm sorry to hear about your father's passing, and can understand why the pain must have bothered you. I need to ask you some specific questions to help me understand the pain a bit better. Is that OK?"*

Empathy. Signposting.

> *Positive CSA indicators*
> - Gathers information efficiently, taking into account the uniqueness of the patient.
> - Gathers information from history taking, examination and investigation in a systematic and efficient manner.

The doctor confirms the diagnosis using closed questions targeted at clarifying a recognisable common condition. These questions do not need to be focused and exhaustive, but the doctor must gather sufficient information to enable them to deal appropriately with the patient's concerns about lymphoma.

> *Positive CSA indicator*
> - Recognises presentation of common problem.

Insufficient evidence	Needs further development	Competent	Excellent
	Generates an adequate differential diagnosis based on the information available.	Makes diagnoses in a structured way using a problem-solving method. Uses an understanding of probability based on prevalence, incidence and natural history of illness to aid decision-making.	Uses pattern recognition to identify diagnoses quickly, safely and reliably. Remains aware of the limitations of pattern recognition and when to revert to an analytical approach.

Positive CSA indicator
- Data gathering appears to be guided by the probabilities of disease.

Doctor: *"How bad has the pain been?"*

The doctor explores the severity of the problem from the patient's perspective. Usually at this point the doctor should have a fair idea of the likely cause and nature of the problem using his knowledge of probability and the natural course of common presentations from the description of the problem by the patient. This early recognition is very useful as it helps the doctor use selective questions that are logical in focusing the rest of the enquiry rather than broad questions used in conventional history taking. This line of enquiry is likely to improve the doctor's insight into the severity of the problem and the impact of the problem on the patient.

Insufficient evidence	Needs further development	Competent	Excellent
From the available evidence, the doctor's performance cannot be placed on a higher point of this developmental scale.	Recognises the impact of the problem on the patient.	Recognises the impact of the problem on the patient, their family and/or carers.	Recognises and shows understanding of the limits of the doctor's ability to intervene in the holistic care of the patient.

Positive CSA indicators
- Explores the impact of the problem.
- Places the problem in the perspective of the uniqueness of the patient.

Patient: *"I've been taking regular anti-inflammatory tablets, which has helped occasionally, but the night times can be a bit of a problem. The pains wake me up a few times when I'm trying to get comfortable, and I have to wake very early in the morning for my job as a taxi driver. It's also become a little bit of a nuisance driving the taxi with it, but it's not something I can't live with as long as I know it isn't anything sinister really. I would have left it a little longer if it wasn't for the fact that I'm going away on a cruise next month, so thought I'd get it checked, especially when it started hurting even when I lift a cup of tea."*

The doctor now understands the impact of the problem and the effects it has on the patient's lifestyle. This information puts the problem in context. A common misunderstanding is that context is the same as social history, but the CSA assesses the relevance of the information the doctor gathers to the patient's problem, and a negative indicator is noted when a doctor asks questions out of context which are perceived as illogical and formulaic. This context gives the doctor an understanding which enables him to find practical and functional solutions to the patient's problem where indicated.

Doctor uses closed questions to clarify his suspicions of a possible soft tissue inflammation, excludes red flags, i.e. systemic features and other joints, completes the drug history, PMH, smoking, etc. The doctor focuses on using questions to exclude any signs of lymphoma to address the patient's concerns.

Doctor: *"I would now like to have a look at the area that is giving you some discomfort – is that OK?"*

Examination: mild tennis elbow, normal elbow movement, and no lymphadenopathies.

Insufficient evidence	Needs further development	Competent	Excellent
	Chooses examination broadly in line with the patient's problem(s).	Chooses examinations appropriately targeted to the patient's problem(s).	Proficiently identifies and performs the scope of examination necessary to investigate the patient's problem(s).

The rest of the consultation is about responding to the doctor's understanding of the uniqueness of the patient using an explanation which demonstrates that understanding, offering options of treatment to respond to the patient's thoughts and preferences, simultaneously showing the connections between the three domains of the CSA.

Doctor: *"The pain is on the part of the outside of the elbow where a group of muscles that control the fingers originate from. This explains why you had pain even when just lifting a cup of tea. The pain can sometimes feel deep in the arm, and may feel like it is in the bone, but the bones don't feel tender to touch at all. I did not feel any lymph nodes in the armpit to suggest anything serious is going on. There are no signs suggesting a lymphoma, and you have said that you feel well in yourself. This condition is sometimes referred to as tennis elbow, just because it's more common from racquet sports like tennis, but can also arise from just using the arm in awkward positions like perhaps putting pressure over that area while driving."*

The doctor explains the problem using his understanding of the patient, to tailor the explanation so as to improve the patient's understanding of the problem. This is an important opportunity for the doctor to 'respond' to his understanding of the patient's perspective. The CSA assesses how the doctor responds to the explored patient's perspective. This response is what links the data gathering and the management decision.

Insufficient evidence	Needs further development	Competent	Excellent
From the available evidence, the doctor's performance cannot be placed on a higher point of this developmental scale.	Provides explanations that are medically correct but doctor-centred.	Uses the patient's understanding to help improve the explanation offered.	Uses a variety of communication techniques and materials (e.g. written or electronic) to adapt explanations to the needs of the patient.

Patient: *"I'm glad you don't think it's in the bone, but is there anything that can be done?"*

Doctor: *"I know you're planning to go on a cruise next month. The anti-inflammatory medication you're taking is useful, and that's why you've noticed some improvement when taking them. I'm not sure whether you would consider trying the same medication but in a cream form, which you can rub directly into the area. This would perhaps mean not having to take the tablets, if that helps."*

The doctor suggests an option, seeking a common ground with the patient, using their knowledge of the management of a common condition.

- Uses an incremental approach, using time and accepting uncertainty.

- Makes plans that reflect the natural history of common problems.

- Offers appropriate and feasible management options.

Insufficient evidence	Needs further development	Competent	Excellent
	Communicates management plans but without negotiating with, or involving, the patient.	Works in partnership with the patient, negotiating a mutually acceptable plan that respects the patient's agenda and preference for involvement.	Whenever possible, adopts plans that respect the patient's autonomy. When there is a difference of opinion the patient's autonomy is respected and a positive relationship is maintained.

Patient: *"I didn't know that the creams might help, but I will give it a go."*

Doctor: *"Normally the point where the muscles attach to the bone would benefit from resting the muscle to reduce the area being pulled, but completely resting the arm would be difficult as I know you have to drive your taxi. Perhaps we could try using a brace to support the elbow and ease the pulling on the area that is inflamed. I'm not sure what you make of this suggestion?"*

Seeking agreement and a common ground.

Patient: *"That would really help, if it will allow me to continue to drive the taxi."*

Doctor: *"If the area is rested, this condition can sometimes resolve within a few weeks on its own without having to do anything further. Occasionally, when it persists, there are other things we can do to resolve it. We may need to consider these options if in the next few weeks it continues to be a problem. I don't think there is any intervention that is likely to resolve the problem for certain before your trip unfortunately, so perhaps it's best if you come back and we can discuss it further after your trip if you're still having problems."*

The doctor can discuss the options of local injection if it appears necessary at this stage, but the management needs to be tailored to the unique situation of the patient to reflect the doctor's understanding of the patient's experience.

Insufficient evidence	Needs further development	Competent	Excellent
	Uses a rigid or formulaic approach to achieve the main tasks of the consultation.	Achieves the tasks of the consultation, responding to the preferences of the patient in an efficient manner.	Appropriately uses advanced consultation skills, such as confrontation or catharsis, to achieve better patient outcomes.

Positive CSA indicators
- Makes a plan that reflects the natural history of the problem.
- Offers feasible options which are tailored to the patient's unique situation.
- Safety netting as appropriate.
- Encourages health promotion where relevant.

This partnership in decision-making is ultimately what the CSA is testing. An ability to achieve this fluently requires practice using the right knowledge of the meaning of the competencies and their application in real life. The CSA is designed to mimic this doctor's real-life performance.

Chapter 10

Offering management options using the patient's understanding

The CSA assesses the ability of the doctor to respond to the patient by demonstrating their understanding of the patient through tailoring the management options they offer to that patient to correspond to their unique situation.[1] In practice most of the doctor's experiences would have involved developing an understanding of the patient's problems more than learning how to understand the patient's experience. It takes more time to perform in this way during the learning stages but quickly becomes efficient when used frequently in practice. With fluency in its use, a doctor becomes more effective and timely by using their understanding of the patient to identify the main tasks of the consultation, making it more focused. Achieving an understanding of the patient's perspectives and gathering clinical information through the perspective of the patient at the same time increases this fluency.[1] This approach is useful because it makes it possible for the doctor to provide the patient with treatment options which are feasible and relevant to their experience of the problem.

The dialogue below demonstrates how the doctor uses their understanding of the patient to tailor the advice and treatment that they offer to the patient.

37-year-old woman

Patient: *"It's my back doctor. It's gone out of sync and I'm struggling to stand straight. It almost feels like my back is rotated out of the centre. I've been dosing myself up with painkillers today, but thought I'd come and get you to have a look."*

The first task is to clarify the reason for attending. This doesn't simply mean the patient's symptoms, but what they have made of the problem that caused them to attend. One patient may attend because they felt the pain is unusual for them and want to know why or whether it is perhaps something serious, and another patient may attend because they want to be signed off from work because they suspect the pain has got something to do with their new job.

The doctor chooses a reflective question that is exploratory enough to encourage the patient to share their experience of the problem. It is within this patient's experience that the doctor gains insight into the reason for attending, and the nature of the decision the patient has attended to make. Achieving a clarification early focuses the rest of the consultation to the main tasks, and gives the doctor an opportunity to be selective in their choice of questions. Every patient is different, and the way everyone feels and thinks about their problems is different. This uniqueness should be discovered early in the consultation using exploratory open questions.

Doctor: *"Can you tell me what has happened exactly?"*

The doctor recognises the need in this case to explore the patient's own account of the problem. The patient's account of the problem will provide the doctor with an opportunity to gain insight into the patient's experience of the problem using active listening and an awareness of verbal cues. The focus at this stage should be on developing a relationship with the patient based on understanding their point of view. This can be done either by gathering data on the nature of the clinical problem from the patient's experience of it, or by exploring the patient's interpretation through encouraging their contribution.

Insufficient evidence	Needs further development	Competent	Excellent
	Develops a relationship with the patient, which works, but is focused on the problem rather than the patient.	Explores and responds to the patient's agenda, health beliefs and preferences. Elicits psychological and social information to place the patient's problem in context.	Incorporates the patient's perspective and context when negotiating the management plan.

Focusing mainly on the clinical problem from the onset of the consultation is unlikely to build the relationship required for the doctor to understand the patient's experience, and would impede the opportunity for the doctor to work in partnership with the patient.

Patient: *"I've suffered with my back for a few years now. I saw the orthopaedic doctors 3 months ago and had an MRI, and they said it was mainly wear and tear. They didn't think there was any need for surgery or anything and I had sessions of physio which helped. I have been OK for the last 2 months but yesterday I felt the back go as I tried to lift a heavy box. It's eased up a little now, but I didn't know for sure whether I should rest it or keep moving."*

The doctor needs to explore the patient's experience and understanding of the events. This will give the doctor more insight into the reason for their attendance. This clarification is important as it allows the doctor to gather information efficiently, taking into account the patient's reason for attending, and to be selective in their choice of enquiries.

> **Positive CSA indicators**
> - Clarifies the problem and nature of decision required.
> - Uses an incremental approach, using time and accepting uncertainty.
> - Gathers information efficiently, taking into account the uniqueness of the patient.
> - Is selective in the choice of the enquiries.

Insufficient evidence	Needs further development	Competent	Excellent
	Accumulates information from the patient that is mainly relevant to their problem. Uses existing information in the patient records.	Systematically gathers information, using questions appropriately targeted to the problem without affecting patient safety. Understands the importance of, and makes appropriate use of, existing information about the problem and the patient's context.	Expertly identifies the nature and scope of enquiry needed to investigate the problem, or multiple problems, within a short time-frame. Prioritises problems in a way that enhances patient satisfaction.

Doctor: *"Does it feel the same as it felt in previous flare-ups?"*

Patient's understanding.

The doctor uses a reflective question to understand the patient's interpretation of the current problem. These types of probing question gives the patient an opportunity to express their inner thoughts about their understanding of the problem. This question was chosen with the aim of inviting the patient to share their thoughts. This is important for the doctor to put the problem and complaint in context.

Patient: *"It does, but the only difference is that this is the first time my back has seized. That worried me a bit as normally I get the pain, but the back doesn't seize. This was why I wondered about whether it would be best to rest it, because doctors always advise you to "move as much as you can". I'm not getting any pains down my legs at all, as I read that it would normally suggest that a nerve is being pinched."*

Patient's thoughts and concerns.

> **Positive CSA indicator**
> - Explores patient's agenda, health beliefs and preferences.

Doctor: *"It sounds like it has been quite bad this time."*

The doctor clarifies the severity of the problem from the patient's point of view using an exploratory statement in the right context. The doctor gains an understanding of the impact of the problem on the patient. The way a problem has affected a patient influences their expectation and reasons for attending and should be understood, as this influences the focus of the rest of the consultation, giving the doctor an opportunity to respond to that understanding when they are offering advice or management options to the patient.

> **Positive CSA indicators**
> - Explores the impact of the illness on the patient's life.
> - Elicits psychological and social information to place the patient's problem in context.

Patient: *"It's actually not been too bad today, but it was quite nasty yesterday. I just couldn't do anything or get comfortable. My main worry is my job. I work in a school as a cleaner, and I doubt I would be able to get into work this week. I've already called the school and they were ever so nice and supportive. I think I can cope as long as I know the best course of action to take."*

The doctor understands the context of the patient's attendance and their experience. Patient's concerns.

Doctor: *"I will ask you some specific questions to help me understand the problem a bit better."*

Signposting. The doctor proceeds to complete their agenda, which is to clarify the suspected diagnosis by focusing on the most likely causes, excluding red flags, specifically confirming the nature of the spasm which concerned the patient, and exclude systemic problems. Have a look at the 'data gathering' competency table. The doctor is expected to gather information targeted to the recognised problem without affecting the patient's safety. This requires a knowledge of the common aetiology of conditions, and an ability to identify patterns of disease using the patient's own description. Closed questions are used to clarify the presence of signs to support the suspected diagnosis, and also to exclude red flags. It is a negative indicator in the CSA for the doctor to use an exhaustive approach in making a diagnosis without showing a systematic approach using their recognition of the problem, and accepting uncertainties.

Insufficient evidence	Needs further development	Competent	Excellent
From the available evidence, the doctor's performance cannot be placed on a higher point of this developmental scale.	Generates an adequate differential diagnosis based on the information available.	Makes diagnoses in a structured way using a problem-solving method. Uses an understanding of probability based on prevalence, incidence and natural history of illness to aid decision-making. Addresses problems that present early and/or in an undifferentiated way by integrating all the available information to help generate a differential diagnosis. Uses time as a diagnostic tool.	Uses pattern recognition to identify diagnoses quickly, safely and reliably. Remains aware of the limitations of pattern recognition and when to revert to an analytical approach.

Negative CSA indicators
- Data gathering does not appear to be guided by the probabilities of disease.
- Does not use an incremental approach.

Doctor: *"Is it OK if I have a look at your back now?"*

Examination: lower lumbar muscle spasm. No spinous process tenderness. Normal neurology. Temp NAD. The choice of examination should be selective enough to verify the doctor's suspicion, exclude red flags and address the patient's concerns.

Positive CSA indicator
- Is appropriately selective in the choice of enquiries, examinations and investigations.

Insufficient evidence	Needs further development	Competent	Excellent
	Chooses examination broadly in line with the patient's problem(s).	Chooses examinations appropriately targeted to the patient's problem(s).	Proficiently identifies and performs the scope of examination necessary to investigate the patient's problem(s).

Diagnosis: non-specific lower back pains with no complications.

Doctor: *"From the examination, I think you're right about the muscle being stiff around the lower back. I know you were concerned about your back seizing up, but it can happen when the muscles go into spasm because of the jarring of the joints of the lower back – perhaps it might have happened at the time you felt your back go. There are no signs to suggest a nerve has been pinched as all the muscles and nerves in your legs are OK, and this would normally give an indication of any problems. It's more likely that it is muscles going into spasm that has made your back seize and caused you to feel out of sync."*

The doctor is explaining the problem using their understanding of the patient's experience in a way that is relevant to the patient and more understandable. It is important to understand that this competency is not simply about using non-jargon in the explanation but rather should reflect the doctor's knowledge of the patient's level of understanding. For instance, it is appropriate to use medical jargon when the patient is a doctor. What is more important is that the explanation given reflects the understanding and the language of the patient to improve the patient's understanding of the information that is being offered.

Insufficient evidence	Needs further development	Competent	Excellent
From the available evidence, the doctor's performance cannot be placed on a higher point of this developmental scale.	Provides explanations that are medically correct but doctor-centred.	Uses the patient's understanding to help improve the explanation offered.	Uses a variety of communication techniques and materials (e.g. written or electronic) to adapt explanations to the needs of the patient.

Positive CSA indicators
- Provides explanations that are relevant and understandable to the patient.
- Responds to needs and concerns with interest and understanding.

Doctor: *"I know you had wanted to discuss the best way to manage the flare-up, but I'm not sure what painkillers you're already taking."*

Seeking common ground. Encouraging contribution by foreseeing the nature of decision using their knowledge of management of common presentations.

Patient: *"I'm alright for painkillers; I have tramadol already, and it's helping."*

Patient's preference discovered through continued encouragement to be involved in decision-making.

Doctor: *"You did say you weren't sure whether it's better for you to keep moving or to rest? I know your movement has been limited by the spasm, but there are tablets we can use to help with the spasms, especially when they're quite bad."*

The doctor uses their knowledge of the management of acute back muscle spasm to focus the discussion and the interventions offered, using their understanding of the patient. This is different from making a list of recommendations without taking into account the circumstances and views of the patient.

Patient: *"Yes, I had some of those the last time, and they are really helpful."*

> *Positive CSA indicators*
> - Makes plans that reflect the natural history of common problems.
> - Offers appropriate and feasible management options.

Doctor: *"It's difficult to move around when the back is seized, but it's usually more beneficial to try as much as you can to get around and stretch the back to avoid the area getting stiff. I'm hoping the spasm tablets would help reduce the spasm so you could move a little easier."*

The doctor is using incremental steps to suggest options of treatment best suited to the unique experience of the problem by the patient to show responsiveness to the patient's views as a partner in the deliberation. The doctor is not offering all the list of options of treatment of back pain to the patient, but using their understanding of the patient's context to tailor the advice.

> *Positive CSA indicators*
> - Shows responsiveness to the patient's preferences, feelings and expectations.
> - Responds to needs and concerns with interest and understanding.
> - Uses an incremental approach, using time and accepting uncertainty.

Doctor: *"I know you said you've had some physiotherapy in the past – are you aware of the type of exercises that might help?"*

The doctor is varying their offer of choice to the patient, using their understanding of the patient and their knowledge of the natural history of the problem. This approach empowers the patient and encourages self-sufficiency.

Insufficient evidence	Needs further development	Competent	Excellent
	Uses appropriate but limited management options without taking into account the preferences of the patient.	Varies management options responsively according to the circumstances, priorities and preferences of those involved.	Provides patient-centred management plans whilst taking account of local and national guidelines in a timely manner.

Patient: *"I feel more reassured now to start doing the stretches. Hopefully the spasm tablets will make it easier."*

Decisions should be made through a partnership by suggesting feasible options, giving the patient an opportunity to continue to share their views. It is important to understand that every individual should be given a chance to make choices related to their health and the doctor should not inappropriately allow their views to influence the dialogue, and should demonstrate respect for the patient's views.

Positive CSA indicators
- Works in partnership, finding common ground to develop a shared management plan.
- Demonstrates respect for others.
- Does not allow own views/values to inappropriately influence dialogue.

Negative CSA indicators
- Instructs the patient rather than seeking common ground.
- Fails to empower the patient or encourage self-sufficiency.

Doctor: *"I think for now, we'll watch and see how you progress with the spasm tablets and some exercises. If you're not getting any relief from the spasm, you should let me know, or if you feel the pain relief you've got already isn't helping. I would expect things to settle within the next 4 to 6 weeks, but you should notify me if you notice any changes, especially if you feel any numbness or weakness in the legs or notice any other changes that concern you."*

If a particular option is not feasible to the patient, or the doctor's understanding is that an option will go against the patient's preference, then it is not necessary to offer every patient all the possible options, as long as patient safety is considered.

Positive CSA indicators
- Uses an incremental approach, using time and accepting uncertainty.
- Makes plans that reflect the natural history of common problems.

Negative CSA indicator
- Does not suggest how the problem might develop or resolve.

Insufficient evidence	Needs further development	Competent	Excellent
	Suggests intervention in all cases.	Considers a "wait and see" approach where appropriate. Uses effective prioritisation of problems when the patient presents with multiple issues.	Empowers the patient with confidence to manage problems independently, together with knowledge of when to seek further help.

Safety net is useful in demonstrating the doctor's awareness of the uncertainties involved in focusing consultations on a patient's problem within the limited time provided, without affecting the patient's safety. The clinical diagnosis should be made based on probability, likelihood and knowledge of the natural course of the condition. To achieve this level of performance, the doctor needs to practise how to manage real-life encounters using this approach.

Doctor: *"I'm wondering what you feel would be the best way to manage the situation at work – I know that you've been off work this week."*

The doctor continues to offer options in a suggestive way, recognising the value of the partnership in decision-making. This does not mean that the doctor should accept everything the patient says, but it gives the doctor an idea of the thoughts of the patient to avoid discordance and enhance compliance.

Negative CSA indicators
- Instructs the patient rather than seeking common ground.
- Uses a rigid approach to consulting that fails to be sufficiently responsive to the patient's contribution.
- Works in partnership, finding common ground to develop a shared management plan.

Patient: *"I'm hoping that with the exercises and medication, I'll be able to go back into work after the weekend. For now, I'd prefer not to take any time off from work unless I feel that I won't be able to cope, and I will certainly let you know."*

Patient feels empowered to contribute to discussion regarding management.

Doctor: *"I agree with you that it will be more beneficial for you to get back to your normal routines as soon as you can, but it would be sensible to avoid lifting heavy objects or doing any strenuous activity for now to avoid aggravating the area further – but continue doing the stretching exercises."*

Shared decision is even more important when the intervention or decision to be made surrounds the patient's own life or lifestyle, as they will need to play an even greater role in making those decisions. Statements like "I'm not sure if you feel there are areas in your diet that perhaps we may be able to improve" are more likely to give the patient an opportunity to participate actively in decisions regarding an important part of their life. The doctor is more likely to get a realistic idea of the motivation of the patient for change. This is different from 'instructing a patient', for example "You need to eat more fruit and vegetables". In the first example, the patient might suggest perhaps cutting down on the sandwiches they eat every lunch time and replacing the bar of chocolate with an apple, but in the second example, the patient answers in the affirmative. When management is offered in a way that is relevant and feasible to the patient, they are more likely to comply with those options, especially if they are part of the decision-making.

Positive CSA indicators
- Encourages improvement, rehabilitation and, where appropriate, recovery.
- Shows responsiveness to the patient's preferences, feelings and expectations.
- Enhances patient autonomy.
- Offers appropriate and feasible management options.

Negative CSA indicator
- Fails to empower the patient or encourage self-sufficiency.

Chapter 11

Dealing with a specialist clinical problem using patient-centredness

The perception that CSA cases are different from real-life patients is not uncommon, but the CSA cases are calibrated to contain the details that the exam is designed to assess, and are more likely to be full of details of the patient's perspective. These details make the approach recommended in this book even more rewarding to use if they are learnt through practice rather than by a formulaic preparatory structure, which is considered a negative indicator in the grading of the CSA, as the doctor is expected to show a genuine interest in developing a therapeutic relationship with the patient. The CSA assesses this relationship with the patient throughout the three domains graded.

Role players used in the CSA share their feelings and thoughts as real patients would do, but only if the questions are asked in the right context, with logical intentions and empathy. A case can only be considered as challenging if the focus of the doctor is on the clinical problem, as regardless of the complexity of the clinical problem presented, the doctor is able to develop a therapeutic relationship with the patient, understand the patient's experience of the problem, empathise and develop rapport with the patient, understand the impact of the problem, clarify their reasons for attending and recognise the clinical condition presented. This will then give the doctor an idea of the exact nature of the decision they have attended to make, focusing the consultation so that the doctor can suggest functional solutions using problem solving that are relevant and feasible.

In the case below, the doctor uses their broad knowledge to guide the patient through the decision-making by problem solving, and understanding the patient's experience.

> **43-year-old woman, married with two children. Known MS patient. Diagnosed 3 years ago. Seen in the neurology clinic recently. She presents today with urinary difficulties.**

Patient: *"I've been struggling with the urge to pass urine for a while now, and I thought I'd get your opinion on how to manage it."*

The doctor listens actively to understand the direction of the patient's thoughts and the purpose of attending to discover the exact nature of the decision the patient has attended to make. She suffers a long-term condition for which she would probably have been seeing a specialist doctor and possibly will have a good awareness of the condition through her experience of it. In this situation the patient's ideas and thoughts play an even bigger role in decision-making.

Doctor: *"It sounds like you're considering specific options."*

Reflective question. The doctor clarifies the reason for attending and the task ahead using an open statement to encourage the patient to share her thoughts. This understanding puts her request into the perspective of her experience, improving the doctor's insight into the reason for attending. The patient's thoughts and views may give the doctor some ideas about her preferences and expectations.

> **Positive CSA indicators**
> - Clarifies the problem and the nature of the decision required.
> - Gathers information efficiently, taking into account the uniqueness of the patient.
> - Places the problem in the perspective of the uniqueness of the patient.
> - Explores the patient's perspective.

Patient: *"I saw the MS nurse yesterday, and she was ever so nice. I discussed the problem with her, and she recommended seeing you to get some tablets to help control the urge to go. She has already given me a mattress protector and some pads, but was unable to prescribe any medications. I've managed the waterworks on my own really well for some time, but I have a wedding to attend next month and I wouldn't want to embarrass myself there."*

Reason for attending. The nature of the decision to make. Patient's expectations.

> **Positive CSA indicator**
> - Explores patient's agenda, health beliefs and preferences.

Doctor: *"I can understand how that must feel, but did she tell you what the medication is?"*

Empathy. Exploring patient's understanding. Focused and logical data gathering.

Trying to identify what the main issues are and the reason for attending. The doctor continues to focus on building a relationship with the patient, but should focus on understanding the patient rather the clinical problem at this stage.

Insufficient evidence	Needs further development	Competent	Excellent
	Develops a relationship with the patient, which works, but is focused on the problem rather than the patient.	Explores and responds to the patient's agenda, health beliefs and preferences. Elicits psychological and social information to place the patient's problem in context.	Incorporates the patient's perspective and context when negotiating the management plan.

Patient: *"She said the tablets might help the bladder gain some control, so it won't be over-reactive. Normally I control my bladder by going every so often just to keep it empty, although they have suggested in the MS clinic that I try self-catheterisation, but I'm reluctant to do that. It will be very difficult on the day of the wedding for me to do that. She didn't specify any particular medication."*

Patient's experience of the situation. Patient's concerns and expectations.

Putting the problem into context, and understanding the impact of the problem. A doctor who has not clarified the reasons for the patient's attendance so far may be distracted by the possible management of a rare condition.

> *Positive CSA indicators*
> - Explores the patient's agenda, health beliefs and preferences.
> - Appears alert to verbal and non-verbal cues.
> - Explores the impact of the illness on the patient's life.
> - Elicits psychological and social information to place the patient's problem in context.

Doctor: *"Did she tell you what might be causing the bladder to behave this way?"*

Clarifying patient's understanding. The doctor will use the patient's understanding as a guide to find common ground for shared decision-making.

Patient: *"She confirmed it was probably due to the MS, but I've had UTIs in the past which can also make the bladder a little more erratic. If it's possible, I would like the urine checked today to make sure there isn't any infection."*

Doctor clarifies the reason for attending, and the nature of the decision to be made.

Patient's thoughts and expectations. Doctor clarifies the tasks through developing an understanding of the patient. The consultation can now be focused appropriately to reflect that insight.

Doctor: *"Can you describe exactly what the symptoms feel like?"*

Using the patient's description to assist the doctor recognise the clinical problem presented and identify the presentation of a common condition. This exploration can be done earlier depending on the individual case presentation and the nature of the task. Data gathered based on a description of the clinical problem can also give the doctor an insight necessary to explore the patient's experience.

Insufficient evidence	Needs further development	Competent	Excellent
	Demonstrates a limited range of data gathering styles and methods.	Demonstrates different styles of data gathering and adapts these to a wide range of patients and situations.	Able to gather information in a wide range of circumstances and across all patient groups (including their family and representatives) in a sensitive, empathetic and ethical manner.

Patient: *"It's not burning when I pass urine, but I don't feel my bladder until it's too late. I could wet myself if I don't make it to the toilet on time. I try to make a mental note of where all the toilets are wherever I go, but this venue is unfamiliar to me. The MS in itself hasn't changed, as they checked me over during my last appointment."*

Understanding the patient's concerns. Gaining insight into the reason for attending. Understanding the impact of the problem, and putting the problem into the right social context.

Doctor uses closed questions to clarify the diagnosis, exclude red flags, drug history and allergies, etc. This focused approach is an important skill in the CSA, which involves the use of selective questions targeted at verifying the likely condition using the knowledge of probability of the disease based on prevalence.

Doctor: *"I'd like to have a look at your tummy and your legs to make sure there aren't any changes."*

Examination: no retention. Temp NAD. No new neurology. urinalysis NAD.

Doctor: *"The urine has no signs of infection, and you're right that it sounds like the kind of changes in the bladder that can be seen in MS."*

The doctor shows responsiveness to their understanding of the patient. They used the explanation to show their understanding of the nature of the decision the patient has attended to make.

Insufficient evidence	Needs further development	Competent	Excellent
From the available evidence, the doctor's performance cannot be placed on a higher point of this developmental scale.	Provides explanations that are medically correct but doctor-centred.	Uses the patient's understanding to help improve the explanation offered.	Uses a variety of communication techniques and materials (e.g. written or electronic) to adapt explanations to the needs of the patient.

Doctor: *"There are a few options of tablets we could consider trying. One of them works by stopping the bladder from being overactive and it is called VESIcare. I don't know if you've heard about this tablet before?"*

Working in partnership. The doctor is suggestive with the offer of treatment, seeking common ground for mutual agreement.

Patient: *"I've read about it very recently on the MS forum, and they're meant to be very good but do have a lot of side effects from what the other members in the forum have reported. There is a medication called desmopressin that a lot of people have found very useful."*

Patient continues to make contributions due to the nature of approach the doctor is using to consult. The consultation is open and inclusive but focused on the task. The patient's perspective does not need to all be explored or realised at once, as the patient may have ideas about treatments etc. as well.

Positive CSA indicators
- Is cooperative and inclusive in approach.
- Uses an incremental approach, using time and accepting uncertainty.

Doctor: *"Desmopressin works a little differently from the tablets that relax an overactive bladder. They are also effective in controlling urine volume but they don't necessary stop the bladder from feeling like it needs emptying often. They also have some side effects, just like the bladder relaxing tablets."*

Insufficient evidence	Needs further development	Competent	Excellent
	Uses a rigid or formulaic approach to achieve the main tasks of the consultation.	Achieves the tasks of the consultation, responding to the preferences of the patient in an efficient manner.	Appropriately uses advanced consultation skills, such as confrontation or catharsis, to achieve better patient outcomes.

Patient: *"That makes sense, it does sound like perhaps I should try these bladder tablets."*

Patient's preference. Empowered to make decisions due to openness of the consultation.

Doctor: *"These tablets are generally safe and used quite often, but the most common side effects are things like constipation and dryness of the mouth. Overall they're effective in controlling the overactive bladder. They're taken once a day, but usually have to be taken every day. They can take a few days or perhaps up to a week to begin to have some effects, but if you have any problems with them, we can review the decision and perhaps consider other alternative tablets. It's also important to continue the bladder training that the MS nurses had advised, and maybe you could let me know within 2 weeks how you get on with the tablets."*

Patient: *"OK."*

Chapter 12

Discovering the reason for a patient's attendance

The dialogue below demonstrates how to discover the reasons for the patient's attendance by encouraging their contribution early in the consultation, and at the same time understanding and recognising the nature of the clinical problem presented by the patient. In the CSA, the doctor is expected to clarify the nature of the issue that the patient has attended to resolve so that the data gathering can be focused on the main issues and tasks of the consultation. It is a negative indicator for the doctor to make an immediate assumption about the problem or use a line of enquiries that is not guided by the probability of the condition being present. Without sufficiently exploring the patient's experience, the doctor is likely to be too broad with their data gathering, which makes it difficult for them to clarify the nature of the decision required in that consultation. Two patients that presented with the same clinical condition can have different reasons for attending, regardless of the fact that the management of the condition may be the same, but the management plan offered needs to be relevant and feasible to the particular circumstances of the patient.

41-year-old man on perindopril 2 mg (BP 145/90 mmHg; cholesterol 5.7)

Patient: *"I really just wanted a check-up. I was told last month that I needed to take tablets for my blood pressure by one of the doctors following a routine check in the surgery. He said my BP has been raised on a few occasions, and recommended that I go on these tablets. I'm not entirely sure what I'm supposed to do next as I've now completed the month's course of the tablets."*

Using active listening, the doctor focuses on understanding why the patient has returned, whether they were asked to return, or what their understanding of the treatment was. Making an immediate assumption of their reason for attending here is likely to cause the doctor to focus on an area that may not be relevant to the patient's reason for attending. The doctor should use reflective questions to encourage the patient to share their thoughts and feelings, as within this context they can gain an insight into the patient's reasons for attending and their perspectives.

Positive CSA indicators
- Clarifies the problem and nature of the decision required.
- Uses an incremental approach, using time and accepting uncertainty.

Negative CSA indicator
- Makes immediate assumptions about the problem.

Doctor: *"How are you getting on?"*

Reflective question aimed at encouraging the patient's contribution. The doctor seeks to explore the patient's thoughts and feelings about the situation with an open question. The doctor chooses to understand the patient visit through their own account of their experience to gain more insight into their views and thoughts. Achieving this insight in this section of the consultation is important as the doctor is able to focus the rest of the consultation using this understanding. It is important to note that questions which are not open enough to encourage the patient's contribution are likely to disrupt the patient from their train, for example "How long have you had the tablets for?" This question is focused on the problem and may deviate the thoughts of the patient to the clinical problem rather than their experience of the problem.

> *Positive CSA indicators*
> - Explores the patient's agenda, health beliefs and preferences.
> - Appears alert to verbal and non-verbal cues.
>
> *Negative CSA indicator*
> - Does not inquire sufficiently about the patient's perspective/health understanding.

Patient: *"I feel very well on the tablets, but I'm not sure if they're really making any difference as I've always been a very anxious person. I get anxious about everything and have been like that for nearly all my life. I've learnt how to control my anxiety a great deal from the therapies that I've had over the years, especially using meditation. I've coped really well by using all the skills and techniques I've learnt to keep myself much calmer and well."*

Doctor: *"It sounds like things are a bit more settled now."*

Empathy. Rapport increases. Explores a verbal cue using paraphrasing.

Checking patient's understanding. Finding common ground. Excluding red flags: anxiety (doctor's agenda).

Patient: *"I learnt a lot from 'mindfulness' classes, and have applied a lot of it in my job to cope with the stresses of every day. There's no problem from that point of view."*

Doctor clarifies that there are no issues of concern from the past history of anxiety.

Doctor: *"What job is it that you do?"*

Opportunistic enquiry. Put the patient's situation in context. In the CSA the doctor is not expected to ask the patient every single question possible about their condition, as long as the doctor demonstrate a logical approach using a line of enquiry which suggests a reasonable focus on understanding the patient's problem and the patient's experience of the problem, without affecting the patient's safety. For instance, asking a question like "How is your diet?" is out of context and in a bid to score points is likely to be considered as a disjointed and unstructured consultation (read the RCGP published reasons for failure feedback). Opportunities occur in the consultation through encouraging the patient's contribution for the doctor to gain insight into the social and psychological context of the problem, as in this case. Patients live and exist in a society, and their experience of a problem should be seen in that context. This enhances a genuine understanding of the impact of the problem, and determines how effective it will be for the doctor to negotiate any management plan with the patient or find a practical solution to their problem.

Insufficient evidence	Needs further development	Competent	Excellent
	Makes decisions by applying rules, plans or protocols.	Thinks flexibly around problems, generating functional solutions.	No longer relies on rules or protocols but is able to use and justify discretionary judgement in situations of uncertainty or complexity, for example in patients with multiple problems.

Positive CSA indicator
- Elicits psychological and social information to place the patient's problem in context.

Patient: *"I'm a computer analyst, and work in my dad's company with my wife. It's a stressful job, but nothing out of the ordinary. I've been able to learn how to balance work and life through a recent course I attended, which was arranged by the therapist. I feel that life cannot get any better than this."*

Doctor gains more insight into the patient's context.

The most efficient way to understand the patient's problem within the context of their life is through using an open question aimed at allowing the patient to share their experience, especially when that question refers to severity or impact. This is different from asking a patient "Are you married?" or "Do you have children?" just as a routine question to help establish the context of the problem, especially when the question appears to be out of context to the natural flow of the consultation. The doctor should be guided by the logical usefulness of the information they gather, and not just a search for every answer.

Doctor: *"What was your understanding from your last consult regarding the tablets?"*

Doctor proceeds to check the patient's understanding. Finding common ground for decision-making. Patient's preference. Previous similar experiences or previous encounters with professionals are a good source of understanding and health beliefs for patients. Doctor seeks to make use of already known information. The doctor is not able to work in partnership with the patient without gaining a sufficient understanding of the patient's experience.

Positive CSA indicators
- Explores the patient's agenda, health beliefs and preferences.
- Appears alert to verbal and non-verbal cues.

Patient: *"The doctor mentioned about a review after a month, at which point we would decide how to proceed. I asked him if I was going to be on the tablets for life, and he indicated that was very likely. The tablets are not bothering me really and I know anxiety can affect blood pressure, as my blood pressure is always on the high side whenever I feel anxious. I'm not sure if perhaps the anxiety might have something to do with the blood pressure – or the other way around."*

Verbal cues. Patient's health beliefs, concerns. Patient's understanding and experience. The patient account of the situation gives the doctor an insight into the reason for their visit. The doctor has focused on developing a relationship with the patient based on understanding their feelings and thoughts about their experience so far.

> **Negative CSA indicators**
> - Does not inquire sufficiently about the patient's perspective/health understanding.
> - Pays insufficient attention to the patient's verbal and non-verbal communication.

Doctor: *"Do you feel perhaps your blood pressure would have been better if it was checked when you were more relaxed?"*

Responding to verbal cues.

Clarifying patient's ideas. Finding common ground.

Patient: *"I've been monitoring it at home since then, and it has remained around 140/70 mmHg. It does go up to around 165 to 170 when I haven't taken the tablets, so I'm sure the tablets are definitely working. I've been taking it regularly for that reason, because I understand the consequences of high blood pressure if it's left untreated. Doing exercises has helped my anxiety a lot, but I must say I haven't been confident to do as much exercise as I would have done since I started the tablets. I wasn't sure if it would be safe to do so as I try to keep very healthy with my general health after the doctor mentioned about my cholesterol being slightly raised as well."*

Patient's experience of the problem. The decisions the patient has attended to make become clearer through an understanding of the patient's perspective. Health beliefs. Finding common ground for decision-making. The insight gained by the doctor will be useful in the decision-making to achieve a mutual agreement, as both parties' views are likely to be taken into account.

Doctor: *"It sounds like you're convinced the tablets have helped, but not sure whether anything else might be impacting on the blood pressure."*

Clarifying the task using summarising.

Patient: *"I wasn't sure if it was possible for someone on blood pressure tablets to stop them if the blood pressure improves with control of my anxiety and perhaps lifestyle changes. I don't mind if I have to take the tablets, although I would like to control it without needing tablets in the future."*

Clarifies the reason for the patient's attendance. The nature of the decision the patient has attended to make. This understanding focuses the consultation to the main task which the patient has attended to resolve.

> *Positive CSA indicators*
> - Clarifies the problem and nature of the decision required.
> - Uses an incremental approach, using time and accepting uncertainty.
> - Gathers information from history taking, examination and investigation in a systematic and efficient manner.
> - Is appropriately selective in the choice of enquiries, examinations and investigations.

Doctor: *"I'd like to ask you some specific questions to understand your general health."*

The doctor clarifies the patient's general health, lifestyle, smoking, alcohol and FH. Excludes red flags, i.e. chest pains and headache.

Signposting. Focused closed question to complete doctor's agenda. CVD risk.

Doctor: *"I'd like to measure your blood pressure – is that alright?"*

Examination: BP 131/82 mmHg, BMI 23.

Focused examination on the problem.

Doctor: *"Your blood pressure is well controlled now, and the readings are similar to what you've been getting at home when you checked while on the tablets. As you know, there are lots of benefits to keeping the blood pressure under control. This benefit continues as long as the blood pressure remains controlled, and it's good that your blood pressure has remained much better than it was before you started the tablets, especially when you're also tolerating the tablet well. The reading you get at home without the tablets does suggest that you're better off on them than not."*

Explanation offered enhanced by using the patient's understanding. The doctor responds to their understanding of the patient in the language they are using. Reinforces the positives.

Insufficient evidence	Needs further development	Competent	Excellent
From the available evidence, the doctor's performance cannot be placed on a higher point of this developmental scale.	Provides explanations that are medically correct but doctor-centred.	Uses the patient's understanding to help improve the explanation offered.	Uses a variety of communication techniques and materials (e.g. written or electronic) to adapt explanations to the needs of the patient.

> *Positive CSA indicators*
> - Shows responsiveness to the patient's preferences, feelings and expectations.
> - Enhances patient autonomy.
> - Provides explanations that are relevant and understandable to the patient.

Doctor: *"I know you'd wondered about the prospects of stopping the tablets at some point. You're right about the effect of anxiety and stress on blood pressure, and the progress you made in learning how to relax more will definitely help your blood pressure. The changes you're making in your lifestyle will also help a lot. Exercising is safe on these tablets, and should help control your blood pressure and the cholesterol without causing you any problems. The most important thing is to keep the pressure within the normal level, no matter how* *we achieve that. Some people might need to be on the tablets for longer than others, depending on how their blood pressure changes on regular monitoring, which is why we recommend yearly reviews. Someone's blood pressure can become so controlled that they can discontinue the tablet, especially if they make the kind of lifestyle changes that you're doing. Assuming you continue to control your anxiety as you are with the exercises, it's possible that we may decide to try without the tablets to see how the blood pressure has responded. How does that sounds to you?"*

Opportunistic health promotion. Addressing the main task. Doctor achieves the task by working in partnership with the patient; that partnership was achieved here by using the patient's understanding in tailoring the advice given to the uniqueness of the patient's experience.

Insufficient evidence	Needs further development	Competent	Excellent
	Uses a rigid or formulaic approach to achieve the main tasks of the consultation.	Achieves the tasks of the consultation, responding to the preferences of the patient in an efficient manner.	Appropriately uses advanced consultation skills, such as confrontation or catharsis, to achieve better patient outcomes.

Patient: *"I'm glad that I can exercise on these tablets, as I read exercise actually helps the blood pressure and the cholesterol. It's also good to know the tablets don't have to be taken forever."*

Mutual understanding. Patient is empowered by the information offered to encourage self-sufficiency. This was achieved because of the doctor's response to their understanding of the patient's experience.

> **Negative CSA indicators**
> - Fails to empower the patient or encourage self-sufficiency.
> - Unable to enhance the patient's health perceptions and coping strategies.

Doctor: *"Perhaps we can review how you're getting on with the changes that you're making in 6 months as you continue with the tablets, to determine how your blood pressure may have responded. From time to time perhaps you could check the reading yourself to help you understand how the effects of the exercise are reflected in the readings. You should notify me if at any time you notice any feelings of light-headedness, especially if the readings are low (less than 100/60 mmHg)."*

Follow-up plan. Safety net.

Chapter 13

Mutually agreed plan using the patient's perspective

The CSA assesses how the doctor gathers data in a way to help them develop an understanding of the clinical problems and also the patient's experience of the problem. The doctor then uses this understanding to seek to find solutions to the patient's problems which are feasible and relevant to their unique situation of the patient, responding to the patient's wishes and preferences. The decisions made during the consultation should be a collaboration between the patient and the doctor on the best options of treatment for the patient. This partnership can only be achieved if both parties are aware of each other's feelings and thoughts about the situation. The doctor's role is to prepare for this negotiation by using a style which encourages the patient to share their inner feelings and being inclusive enough to allow the patient to play a significant role in the decision-making. This is different from when the doctor makes a decision and then seeks to gain the patient's agreement.

To achieve a shared decision, the doctor needs to develop:

1. An ability to recognise a common condition and to know the reasonable, acceptable options of management.

2. Sufficient knowledge of the patient's perspective of the problem.

3. Awareness of the impact of the problem on the patient's life and the context.

The dialogue below explores how to achieve a mutually agreed plan using the patient's perspective.

57-year-old woman (cholesterol 6.8)

Patient: *"I feel well in myself, but had a blood test last week. I had a call from the nurse who asked me to attend to discuss my cholesterol level with you. She said the result was 6.8 and has gone up from the previous year."*

The doctor should actively listen to the patient at this stage, to gain an insight into the patient's reason for attending. She has indicated that she felt well, and was asked to attend. Does she know why? Has she thought about it? What sort of discussion does she want to have? Is she seeking advice or has she made a decision? Does she have questions about the situation? How much is she aware of the interpretation of cholesterol? Does she think the levels reflect her lifestyle? Will she want tablets? Does she know the options? These details will place the situation in the context of the individual patient. These thoughts will reveal the nature of the decision the patient has attended to make, and can only be understood if the doctor is able to efficiently encourage the patient's contribution to the consultation. An experienced doctor will be aware that this understanding may or may not in fact exist, and will approach the consultation with that flexibility in mind. Verbal cues are crucial in exploring the patient's thoughts. Occasionally the doctor may need to proceed with a focus on the problem first, and then build on the patient's experience using communication skills.

The ability to gain an understanding of the patient experience puts the problem in the right context, and allows the consultation to follow a logical structure. The doctor's agenda would be questions like "What is her CVD risk?", "What is her CVS PMH?", "Are there any other causes of the raised cholesterol?", "What is her lifestyle?". These questions are best explored with closed selected questions, but the focus will largely depend on the patient's situation, preferences, previous knowledge, health beliefs, and the decision she has in fact attended to discuss. This understanding is important for the doctor to bear in mind when approaching any consultation. It is almost impossible to rehearse any patient's unique experience, but easier to rehearse the skills required to elicit any patient's perspective of a problem in any circumstance or case. This removes the idea of a 'difficult case'. These understandings put the patient's problem in context, which gives the doctor an opportunity to work in partnership with the patient. The answers to these thoughts in the doctor's mind become more apparent if they are able to use reflective questions through active listening to encourage the patient to share their views freely. Formulaic questions like "What do you think is causing the level to rise?" at this stage might seem a little bit too direct for some patients as they may not have developed enough rapport with the doctor to feel able to share their inner thoughts.

It's clear that the three CSA domains of the assessment are based around the doctor's understanding of the patient rather than a focus on the clinical problem. In fact, if you look closely under 'clinical management', it states that the doctor should be able to recognise the presentation of common problems and offer feasible options rather than learning the detailed management of rare conditions. The CSA cases are designed to mimic the day-to-day encounters of doctors, and the cases are calibrated from real-life encounters as used in this book to capture the uniqueness of the patient's experience. The doctor needs to learn how to recognise and make clinical decisions using probability based on prevalence, and not asking all the questions but being guided by the patient's experience and the nature of their problem.

Positive CSA indicators
- Recognises presentations of common physical, psychological and social problems.
- Uses an incremental approach, using time and accepting uncertainty.

Doctor: *"What did you make of the result?"*

Doctor is checking the patient's understanding. The doctor uses active listening to discover how the patient feels about the result, and the nature of the decision they may have attended to make. The patient's unique experience puts the cholesterol of 6.8 in context. Early clarification of the task of the consultation focuses the consultation on the main issues. It is easy to assume the patient has simply attended to discuss how to bring down the level of her cholesterol, but patients are different as to how they understand, perceive, or prefer to be treated. This individuality of patients is the reason the doctor should not assume what the tasks are, but actively clarify these tasks either by asking directly or more effectively by learning how to explore the patient's perspective of the problem. Within this context the doctor gains insight into the reasons for the patient's attendance.

> *Positive CSA indicator*
> * Clarifies the problem and the nature of the decision required.

Patient: *"Well, I don't know really. I feel well in myself. My husband – who has always had a normal cholesterol level all his life – has recently had a heart attack. I know we're all different, but I have tried statins previously and after 2 days I suffered terrible severe muscle aches. I stopped taking them immediately and have since been working on my cholesterol with diet and exercise."*

Patient's experience puts the result in context almost immediately. The doctor gains understanding of the direction of the patient's thoughts about the situation. The doctor develops insight into the potential nature of the discussion to come, and is able to empathise with the patient more appropriately with the knowledge of their unique experience. This understanding improves rapport. Patient indicates a preference.

Insufficient evidence	Needs further development	Competent	Excellent
	Develops a relationship with the patient, which works, but is focused on the problem rather than the patient.	Explores and responds to the patient's agenda, health beliefs and preferences. Elicits psychological and social information to place the patient's problem in context.	Incorporates the patient's perspective and context when negotiating the management plan.

> *Positive CSA indicators*
> * Explores the patient's agenda, health beliefs and preferences.
> * Explores the impact of the illness on the patient's life.
> * Elicits psychological and social information to place the patient's problem in context.

Doctor: *"So sorry to hear of your husband's heart attack. I can understand what you mean by 'we are all different'. It sounds like you've really tried to keep the levels down, so what do you suspect might be the reason for the level still being high?"*

Empathy, checking the patient's understanding, understanding the patient's thoughts and preferences, gaining insight into the nature of the decision to be made, building rapport, finding common ground for a shared decision, gathering information to assist in giving the patient advice, gathering information to tailor the options offered.

The doctor will only be able to achieve a mutually agreed plan if they are able to foresee those decisions ahead and prepare the common ground through developing an understanding of the position of the other party (the patient) in the negotiation.

Patient: *"I've really been a bit careless with cheese over the last few months, to be honest, as I had thought all the exercises I've been doing recently might have kept the cholesterol under control, but obviously it hasn't really. This is almost like a 'wake-up call' for me to cut the cheese right down, because I'm someone who takes their health very seriously. I love cheese a lot and can go through a 300 g block in a day."*

Patient's preference. Health beliefs. Doctor understands the nature of the decision to be made, and the reason for the patient's attendance, gains insight into the uniqueness of the problem to the patient. Doctor is able to find a practical and functional solution through gaining common ground and the patient's understanding to enhance decision-making. The doctor is gathering information to enhance partnership and improve rapport as the patient feels empowered to share their views.

> **Positive CSA indicator**
> - Works in partnership, finding common ground to develop a shared management plan.

Doctor: *"It sounds like you would prefer to continue working on your diet?"*

Clarifying the task. Checking understanding. Preparing common ground for the task. Establishing the patient's preference.

This understanding will focus the doctor's enquiry to relevant aspects of the consultation.

> **Positive CSA indicator**
> - Clarifies the problem and the nature of the decision required.

Patient: *"I wouldn't like to go back on those horrible tablets if I can avoid it, as I really don't want to relive that pain ever again. I was quite pleased at the time that the pain eased completely and almost immediately after stopping the medication. I will try and work very hard with the diet aspect of it to see what I can achieve before considering any other steps. I don't mind considering any other option that is not simvastatin, as I'm aware of the importance of controlling the cholesterol with regards to heart disease and stroke."*

The patient's agenda is clear. The doctor is able to focus the consultation to the task using their understanding of the patient's agenda. The doctor understands the patient's preference and expectations from the consultation and the decision to be made. The doctor now understands the patient's perspective. The doctor is able to consider a functional solution by the opportunity presented by this approach using problem-solving skills and thinking flexibly around the unique situation of the patient, with empathy increasing rapport.

Insufficient evidence	Needs further development	Competent	Excellent
	Makes decisions by applying rules, plans or protocols.	Thinks flexibly around problems, generating functional solutions.	No longer relies on rules or protocols but is able to use and justify discretionary judgement in situations of uncertainty or complexity, for example in patients with multiple problems.

Doctor's agenda. The doctor uses closed and specific questions to clarify the general health of the patient and takes a brief family history. Personal history of heart problems. Drug history, verifies patient's lifestyle/exercise, alcohol. Smoking to get a view of likely cause of her raised cholesterol. Exclude red flags: alcoholism. Thyroid problems. The choice of question should be logical and should demonstrate an awareness of the probabilities of the condition based on prevalence.

Focused history based on an understanding of the main task. The doctor is also a part of the partnership in the decision-making, and also needs to make sure their thoughts and views are heard and understood by the patient. The doctor should be aware of the risks and be able to share these effectively with the patient, showing a response to their understanding of the patient's health beliefs, concerns, etc.

> *Positive CSA indicators*
> - Gathers information from history taking, examination and investigation in a systematic and efficient manner.
> - Is appropriately selective in the choice of enquiries, examinations and investigations.

The information the doctor has gathered so far is not mainly relevant to the problem, but appropriately targeted to the problem as experienced by the patient.

Examination: BP 120/70 mmHg, CVD risk 7%, BMI 27.

Doctor: *"I agree with you that every individual is different, and you're right about the relationship between the cholesterol levels and the risk of heart disease and stroke. Some people with normal cholesterol can still go on to have a heart attack like you said, but overall we know the lower the level of cholesterol, the lesser the risk in the majority of people. These decisions are best made on an individual basis. I can understand your feelings about the previous simvastatin you tried, and it's probably not a good idea to try that same tablet again. I think your plan of doing more on the diet front is very reasonable, and would encourage your efforts there. It should certainly make a difference."*

Giving information using the patient's understanding of the problem. Responding to patient's understanding and preferences. The response makes the patient feel listened to, enhancing rapport. Information given in this way shows responsiveness to the patient's feelings and preferences. It's important to remember that a patient's preference is not just limited to their choice of treatment, but also the choice of the amount of information they appear willing to engage in, as lecturing a patient who is not really keen on the information may not represent a good responsiveness.

> *Positive CSA indicators*
> - Shows responsiveness to the patient's preferences, feelings and expectations.
> - Enhances patient autonomy.
> - Provides explanations that are relevant and understandable to the patient.

Doctor: *"I'm not sure whether you have any specific guides at home to help you with your diet choices?"*

Finding common ground in decision-making. The doctor suggests options rather than dictating. Finding functional solutions using patient's understanding. Tailoring option to reflect an understanding of the patient's perspective. Varying management options. The doctor avoids discussion on tablets, responding to the patient's preference.

> **Positive CSA indicators**
> • Encourages improvement, rehabilitation and, where appropriate, recovery.
> • Encourages the patient to participate in appropriate health promotion and disease prevention strategies.

Patient: *"My daughter is a dietitian, and she gave me a very useful guide I can use. I believe there are definitely changes I can make in my diet and hopefully that will help. I'll do anything to avoid that horrible medication."*

Mutual agreement.

> **Positive CSA indicator**
> • Works in partnership, finding common ground to develop a shared management plan.

Doctor: *"I know you mentioned about the bad effect you had previously from simvastatin 40 mg. I know you take your health very seriously, but I'm not sure if you were aware that there are different kinds of cholesterol tablets. Someone can react badly to one type of cholesterol tablet but tolerate another type very well, so perhaps it's worth having that in your mind until we review your progress with the diet changes."*

Doctor's agenda.

Giving information to empower the patient but showing responsiveness to the patient's preference. Management option offered as a suggestion, giving an opportunity for the patient to play a significant part rather than prescription and then seeking agreement after decision has been made by the doctor.

> **Negative CSA indicators**
> • Instructs the patient rather than seeking common ground.
> • Uses a rigid approach to consulting that fails to be sufficiently responsive to the patient's contribution.
> • Fails to empower the patient or encourage self-sufficiency.

Patient: *"I didn't know there were other types. I'll probably see what I can achieve with diet in the first instance, but that is actually interesting. Perhaps if the level remains high after making some changes we could consider trying other options."*

Respecting patient's preference. Autonomy.

Insufficient evidence	Needs further development	Competent	Excellent
	Uses a rigid or formulaic approach to achieve the main tasks of the consultation.	Achieves the tasks of the consultation, responding to the preferences of the patient in an efficient manner.	Appropriately uses advanced consultation skills, such as confrontation or catharsis, to achieve better patient outcomes.

Doctor: *"I suggest perhaps checking the cholesterol level again in about 6 months to see what progress you're making."*

Safety net should reflect the doctor's understanding of the patient's concerns, the doctor's agenda and knowledge of the natural course of the condition.

> *Positive CSA indicators*
> - Makes plans that reflect the natural history of common problems.
> - Manages risk effectively, safety netting appropriately.

A doctor may have a broader knowledge of the clinical and pharmacological management of cholesterol but be unable to identify the patient's thoughts, preferences and uniqueness to tailor that knowledge to the patient situation in a safe way. They will then fail to demonstrate patient-centredness, which is what the CSA assesses. The recognition of the patient's perspective puts the patient problems in the context of that patient, and it is in this context that the doctor is assessed to see how fluently they are able to find common ground in a focused way without affecting patient safety.

Chapter 14

Making ethical decisions using patient-centredness

Patient-centredness is even more valuable in cases that present ethical challenges. Doctors make decisions regularly within the context of any consultation to reflect an understanding of how they may have weighed the benefits and the risks of the decisions they make or interventions they offer to the patient. A doctor who practises in a patient-centred manner offers the patient an opportunity to play a major role in this decision-making regarding their own health, to enhance their autonomy. This empowerment is achieved by encouraging the patient's contribution to the consultation, and agreeing a safe and reasonable plan of action using the doctor's knowledge of possibilities and risk tailored to their understanding of the patient's understanding, health beliefs and experiences. Although ethical cases may seem more challenging in the CSA, using the same approach as discussed in this book will provide the doctor with the level of detail of the patient's experience and preferences required to balance the decisions in a way that will respect the patient's autonomy, and also remain safe and within acceptable standards of care. This is the same principle that guides ethical decision-making.

57-year-old woman requesting a referral to the memory clinic

Patient: *"I want a referral to the memory clinic."*

Opening statement. Doctor has no idea of the patient's experience or reason why they have attended. Any assumptions would create discordance and damage rapport.

Doctor: *"Can you tell me why you've decided that you need to be referred to the memory clinic?"*

Reflective question. Doctor uses active listening, showing they heard the patient and are willing to encourage them to share their experience and thoughts using an open question.

Patient: *"My mother was recently diagnosed with dementia, and she had been going to her doctor's for over a year complaining of problems with her memory, but nobody sent her to the memory clinic for investigations because her dementia wasn't obvious. Now it's too late for her, isn't it? I don't want to have to go through the same thing, and would like to get checked now rather than later."*

Patient's concerns and unique experiences. Doctor likely to genuinely empathise. Reason for attending. The doctor needs to clarify the nature of the decision she has attended to make. That reason will explain why she had considered a referral.

Doctor: *"I'm sorry to hear about your mother. I can understand how that must make you feel. Do you have any idea what might happen at the memory clinic?"*

Empathy. Increases rapport. Checking patient's understanding. Finding common ground. Doctor will need to understand to provide information to the patient. This understanding will focus the doctor's data gathering on the task. The doctor is gathering data mostly related to the patient's experience of the problem.

Patient: *"I know the doctors made the diagnosis after my mother had a head scan, so they must have a way of telling from a scan. The questions doctors use in the surgery are not really reliable are they? I remember my mother used to get all the questions right when the doctor asked her those questions about date of birth and so on, but she still ended up with this horrible illness."*

Patient's health beliefs. Patient's understanding clearer. Doctor understands the reason for attending and the nature of the decision to be made without using formulaic questions. Doctor shows willingness to encourage the patient's contribution, improving rapport. Patients are more likely to share their thoughts if they are not interrupted by doctor-centred questions.

Doctor: *"It must have been a horrible time for everyone."*

Empathy. Verbal cue 'horrible'. This is a good way to explore the impact of a problem on a patient's life, by probing into severity. Questions like "How bad has it been?" rather than formulaic questions like "How has this affected you?", which can sometime seem out of context. The doctor suspects an underlying psychological impact. This question likely to put her request into the context of the patient's 'lifeworld'.

Patient: *"My mother brought me up an only child as a single mother, and she gave me everything I have in my life. She's a very strong lady and is fighting the illness, but the last thing I want is not to be there for her, especially now that she's got dementia. That's why I don't want to take any chances. I'd rather get checked even if it means wasting the NHS's money."*

Psychological impact. Patient's concerns.

Doctor: *"Have you noticed any problems with your memory?"*

Data gathering now focused on the problem but the choice of question is more likely to be focused on the doctor's recognition of the problem, and their understanding of the reason for the patient's attendance or concerns. The sequence of the choice of the initial area to probe depends largely on the patient's presentation of the problem, but often the doctor would require an understanding of the patient's problems first, i.e. vague symptoms, worrying symptoms, etc.

> **Negative CSA indicator**
> - Data gathering does not appear to be guided by the probabilities of disease.

Patient: *"Apart from silly things like occasionally forgetting to record a TV programme, I've been fine, but my mother wasn't really that bad with her memory either, and she was still diagnosed with dementia. I haven't noticed any problems at my workplace, and none of the friends I've asked have said there was anything wrong with my memory."*

Patient's ideas. The doctor will respond to this idea during the explanation and advice-giving. Data gathering using the patient's experiences enhances the decision-making, as the doctor is more likely to find common ground for sharing that decision with the patient using that understanding.

> **Positive CSA indicator**
> - Responds to needs and concerns with interest and understanding.

Doctor: *"Did the doctor mention the kind of dementia she was diagnosed with?"*

Finding common ground. Doctor is aware of focused data necessary to achieve the task identified. Failure to identify the task will not give the doctor the focus they need to address the patient's task, causing discordance during the decision-making. If the doctor does not gain insight into the patient's understanding, it will be difficult to build rapport.

Patient: *"The doctor said it was vascular dementia from the dots on the scan."*

Doctor: *"I'm not sure what you understand about the types of dementia?"*

Checking understanding, finding common ground.

> **Positive CSA indicator**
> - Works in partnership, finding common ground to develop a shared management plan.

Patient: *"Not a lot, but my mother can't stop reminding me to get checked, I suspect it runs in families I guess."*

Patient's health beliefs and understanding. The doctor uses the information to tailor and improve the explanation and advice they offer the patient, enhancing rapport further. Doctor uses the information to work in partnership with the patient. The patient is empowered through the doctor's understanding of their own thoughts. Inability to explore the patient's health beliefs will mean the doctor is unable to empower the patient effectively or enhance those beliefs.

> **Negative CSA indicator**
> - Unable to enhance patient's health perceptions and coping strategies.

Doctor: *"What's the situation right now with you and your mother, do you live together?"*

Support. Functional solutions, impact of the problem. Context is important in finding functional workable solution. The enquiry is guided by the doctor's appreciation of possible causes of problems and in this case, home situation.

Insufficient evidence	Needs further development	Competent	Excellent
	Makes decisions by applying rules, plans or protocols.	Thinks flexibly around problems, generating functional solutions.	No longer relies on rules or protocols but is able to use and justify discretionary judgement in situations of uncertainty or complexity, for example in patients with multiple problems.

Patient: *"She's now moved in with me, as I was worried she may not cope on her own. She is still able to do things for herself, and her dementia is not yet that bad. She's able to go out on her own, for instance, but I know it's definitely a matter of time before she needs all the help she can get. I really want to keep myself healthy to be there for her."*

Health belief, reason for attending, concerns, understanding her preference.

The doctor clarifies the patient's general health. Brief history of lifestyle. Drug history. Smoking.

Closed question. The data required from the patient's history is limited. The doctor recognised an opportunistic health promotion related to vascular diseases.

Doctor: *"I'd like to take your blood pressure and your weight."*

Examination: BP 120/70 mmHg, BMI 22.

Doctor: *"I can understand why you considered a referral to the memory clinic. The question tests we use in the surgery, like you said, only give us an idea about where there is a problem with someone's memory, but the presence of an actual problem with memory is what confirms a problem. Unfortunately, there are no scans available anywhere that can predict the possibilities of dementia in the future. No one would have been able to predict your mother's dementia, as a lot of people may have mini-strokes without developing dementia. The other types of dementia are diagnosed mostly from someone noticing that there was a problem, there is no test available to predict the possibilities of it happening in the future. Although I understand why you felt the memory clinic might be able to tell if you could develop dementia in the future, I wouldn't like to waste your time referring you to it when I know there isn't a test available to help you resolve your question. I'm sure this is disappointing for you, but it may be reassuring for you to know that vascular dementia isn't inherited and there are things we can do to reduce the risk of someone having a mini-stroke in the future."*

The doctor uses their understanding of the patient's thoughts and health beliefs to improve the explanation they offer, addressing the reason for the patient's attendance, addressing the decision the patient has attended to make. The patient came in for a referral, but the decision they wanted to make was to test for chances of future memory impairment. If the doctor failed to explore the patient's experience, she may not have realised the reason behind the request, which can cause a discordance. The doctor addresses the patient's concerns.

Insufficient evidence	Needs further development	Competent	Excellent
From the available evidence, the doctor's performance cannot be placed on a higher point of this developmental scale.	Provides explanations that are medically correct but doctor-centred.	Uses the patient's understanding to help improve the explanation offered.	Uses a variety of communication techniques and materials (e.g. written or electronic) to adapt explanations to the needs of the patient.

Positive CSA indicator
- Provides explanations that are relevant and understandable to the patient.

Patient: *"I'm somewhat relieved to know the vascular dementia she was diagnosed with isn't inherited. You're right, if there is no test available there wouldn't be any use attending the clinic."*

Mutual understanding. The doctor found common ground through developing an understanding of the patient.

Insufficient evidence	Needs further development	Competent	Excellent
	Uses a rigid or formulaic approach to achieve the main tasks of the consultation.	Achieves the tasks of the consultation, responding to the preferences of the patient in an efficient manner.	Appropriately uses advanced consultation skills, such as confrontation or catharsis, to achieve better patient outcomes.

Doctor: *"You're right. There isn't, but there are things one can do to reduce the risk of having a mini-stroke in the future."*

Health promotion.

Doctor: *"I know you exercise twice a week to control your weight; your weight is within the healthy range. That will definitely help reduce your risk of having a heart problem or mini-stroke. You don't smoke, and that on its own also reduces your risk a great deal. The changes you've been making will not only help keep your weight healthy like you said, but also your risk of having a mini-stroke. It's worth knowing that this type of dementia is extremely rare in people of your age."*

Opportunistic positive reinforcement.

Insufficient evidence	Needs further development	Competent	Excellent
	Considers the impact of the patient's lifestyle on their health.	Consistently encourages improvement and rehabilitation and, where appropriate, recovery. Encourages the patient to participate in appropriate health promotion and disease prevention strategies.	Coordinates a team-based approach to health promotion in its widest sense. Maintains a positive attitude to the patient's health even when the situation is very challenging.

Patient: *"That is reassuring."*

Doctor: *"We can still think about taking further action if at any time in the future you notice any problems with your memory. If you also feel that looking after your mother is getting a bit difficult, you can come in and discuss that with me."*

Safety net. Reassurance. Building rapport.

The safety net should reflect the doctor's understanding of the need or the nature of the problem. It should be safe and appropriate whilst enhancing autonomy.

> *Positive CSA indicator*
> - Uses an incremental approach, using time and accepting uncertainty.

Insufficient evidence	Needs further development	Competent	Excellent
	Identifies and tolerates uncertainties in the consultation, but struggles to reassure the patient or to manage it independently.	Is able to manage uncertainty, including that experienced by the patient.	Anticipates and employs a variety of strategies for managing uncertainty.

Chapter 15

Building the history around the patient's experience

There are many consultation models recommending the use of a section of the history taking specifically for collecting data; this is often referred to as ICE (ideas, concerns, expectations). This approach can cause problems in real patient consultations when these ICE questions are misunderstood by the doctor to mean the use of rigid pre-prepared enquiries to explore the patient's perspective, without appreciating the central role patient perspective plays in focusing the rest of the consultation. Patients don't follow a specific structured pattern of behaviour when sharing their thoughts and feelings and are more likely to share those views when explaining their experience of the problem. This is why reflective questioning and active listening are such effective skills in exploring the patient's perspective. Their concerns may be a result of their health beliefs, or their expectation may be as a result of their concerns, for example.

Patient do not always have their ideas, concerns and expectations formulated well and so they often don't understand or respond to standard ICE questions very well in real life, even when they do have concerns and expectations. For example, a patient who presents with piles may be hoping for a referral to a surgeon for banding, having read that suppositories are not effective when the piles are external. But when asked directly whether they have any concerns, they may respond appropriately because they had not considered those thoughts described above as concerns.

Patients respond better when the rapport/relationship is good and the consultation is approached in an inclusive manner to encourage them to share their innermost thoughts rather than respond to interview-style questioning. The doctor will then appreciate the patient's concerns and expectations within the context of them sharing their thoughts and views about the situation.

> *Positive CSA indicator*
> * Is cooperative and inclusive in approach.

These details are best discovered through encouraging the patient to share their own experience of the problem but guided by the doctor using reflective and active listening. The patient's experience and views either become apparent or can be explored through the observation and recognition of verbal and non-verbal cues. Patients may have an opinion about a possible cause of a problem, but may not have considered those views relevant, and are therefore often reluctant to share those views unless they perceive the consultation has been made open enough for them to feel their contributions are valued. This response to the genuine interest and warmth of the doctor is assessed in the CSA, explaining why questions like

"What were you hoping I would do for you today?" often do not provide the robust insight that the doctor requires to sufficiently understand the patient. The most efficient way to achieve an understanding of the clinical problem and develop an understanding of the patient is to gather the history around the patient's experience.

Gathering data using the patient's description of the problem from exploratory questions will achieve both the understanding of the patient's perspective and give the doctor an opportunity to recognise the clinical problem presented. This recognition, rather than exhaustive exploration of the clinical problem, is more efficient and is a positive indicator in the CSA.

Positive CSA indicator
- Recognises the presentations of common physical, psychological and social problems.

The dialogue below demonstrates how data can be gathered from the patient's perspective to recognise the likely diagnosis and also understand the patient's experience of the problem simultaneously.

37-year-old woman

Patient: *"It's my back again, doctor. It's been bad for 2 months now, and I'm struggling to put up with it. I thought perhaps I should talk to you about it, to decide how best to deal with it."*

Using active listening, the doctor understands the patient's frustration. It's clear that the patient has suggested a recurrence of their problem, which has lasted longer than they expected. She is expressing some frustrations about the problem, and considering the best course of action for dealing with the problem.

Listening attentively to the opening statement gives the doctor an idea of the direction of enquiry needed to encourage the patient to share their views, especially in cases that involve an ongoing problem. The first task is to clarify the reason for the patient's attendance and the nature of the decision the patient has attended to make. The patient may have attended to discuss analgesia, a wheelchair service, travel insurance, referral, etc. Clarifying this reason focuses the consultation around the patient's experience of the problem rather than the problem itself, so the tasks of the consultation can be achieved. Subsequently, the identification and recognition of the clinical problem using focused closed enquiry without affecting the patient's safety is the doctor's agenda. This should be done effectively using logical selective questions that demonstrate the doctor's understanding of the probabilities of disease based on prevalence.

Doctor: *"It sounds like you have suffered back pains in the past."*

Questions aimed at establishing the patient's understanding using a verbal cue from the opening statement. This type of question can help the doctor gain an insight into the patient's understanding of their current problem using their previous experience or knowledge of the problem. It is an open question capable of encouraging the patient to share their views and experience.

Insufficient evidence	Needs further development	Competent	Excellent
	Develops a relationship with the patient, which works, but is focused on the problem rather than the patient.	Explores and responds to the patient's agenda, health beliefs and preferences. Elicits psychological and social information to place the patient's problem in context.	Incorporates the patient's perspective and context when negotiating the management plan.

Patient: *"I've suffered from my bad back for so many years. It seems to run in our family as my mother and my two sisters suffer with their backs too. I haven't really seen a doctor about it because it usually resolves within a few days whenever it flares up, but this time has been different and unusual as it has gone on for 2 months. I don't think I've done anything in particular to hurt my back, but I suddenly felt it go as I bent forward to pick something very light up from the floor. It hasn't been giving me problems every day, but some days can be quite awful."*

The doctor gains an insight into the patient's understanding of the problem, and at the same time gains insight into the likely cause of the recent flare-up. They chose the question to develop an understanding of the patient's experience and feelings. The question also reflects the doctor's ability to actively listen. Patients are likely to share their views more freely when they perceive the doctor's willingness to encourage their contribution. This understanding enhances rapport. The information given to the role players in the CSA is designed to reflect this pattern of behaviour and response from the patient. There are details of their experience which the role player will only provide if they feel the doctor has asked the right questions in the right context with genuine interest. Asking "What are your concerns?" after the patient has just said that they haven't had any sleep for 2 weeks, may be seen as an illogical step and unstructured. The doctor should perhaps have first shown empathy and indicated that they understand the patient's take on the situation and perhaps how bad the patient feels the situation has become. Such details are likely to encourage the patient to share their views, including their concerns, or provide verbal cues, which may help the doctor discover their concerns and reasons for attending.

Doctor: *"I wonder what might be the reason for this particular episode lasting longer than usual?"*

Exploring the patient's thoughts and ideas.

Previous experiences and existing information are an important part of the patient's understanding of their problem and their experience. The doctor is not focused mainly on the symptoms but on developing an understanding of the symptom by exploring the patient's experience of the problem.

Insufficient evidence	Needs further development	Competent	Excellent
	Accumulates information from the patient that is mainly relevant to their problem. Uses existing information in the patient records.	Systematically gathers information, using questions appropriately targeted to the problem without affecting patient safety. Understands the importance of, and makes appropriate use of, existing information about the problem and the patient's context.	Expertly identifies the nature and scope of enquiry needed to investigate the problem, or multiple problems, within a short time-frame. Prioritises problems in a way that enhances patient satisfaction.

Patient: *"I don't really know as I've done exactly what I used to do with other episodes. I've been doing back exercises and taken some painkillers. It got a bit better, but yesterday was quite bad. I stayed in bed all day, but have managed to get around today. I suspected probably I wasn't doing the right exercise for this particular episode."*

Patient's thoughts. Reason for attending. Nature of decision to be made. Patient's concerns.

Doctor: *"How bad was it yesterday?"*

Understanding the impact of the problem. Logical opportunity following the line of thought of the patient. Questions related to description of severity from the patient's point of view are useful for understanding the problem and the patient simultaneously. They can put the problem in a real day-to day-context, and it is different from asking "From 1 to 10 where is the pain?"

> *Positive CSA indicators*
> - Explores the impact of the illness on the patient's life.
> - Elicits psychological and social information to place the patient's problem in context.

Patient: *(in tears) It was terrible. I couldn't get comfortable. It's really difficult when you have a 2-year-old to look after with no one to help. I was close to calling the paramedics out last night, it was that bad. That was why I felt maybe this is the right time to get professional guidance, so I don't cause more damage."*

Doctor: *"I'm sorry to hear how difficult it was. Have you considered any options?"*

Checking patient's understanding. Empathy. Reason for patient's attendance is clear. Perspective and context.

Patient: *"I know my mother sees a physiotherapist, which has helped her back a lot. I think maybe it's time to do something more specific to improve the weaknesses in my back. I know there are other invasive treatments for back pain, but I would really prefer to try something like physiotherapy rather than anything invasive if I can avoid it. I thought if you'd had a look, and there isn't any major damage, then I could be referred to see a physiotherapist."*

The doctor understands what the patient thinks about the back pains, gained insight into the severity of the problem, understands why they have attended and what they had planned to achieve. At the same time the doctor has gained an insight into the clinical problem, and probably at this stage made a reasonable diagnostic possibility. The doctor needs to focus the data gathering to the specific problem using their knowledge of possible common causes. Have a look at the 'data gathering' competency recommending 'gathering data' using questions appropriately targeted to the patient and 'adapting data gathering' to the situation and the patient.

> ### Positive CSA indicators
> - Explores the patient's agenda, health beliefs and preferences.
> - Appears alert to verbal and non-verbal cues.

The next stage of the consultation is to clarify the clinical problem, to help the doctor confirm their clinical diagnosis and exclude sinister problems. Using the understanding gained from exploring the patient's perspective, the doctor is able to focus their enquiries, and deal with the patient's concerns. Closed questions are more suited to achieving this task. The description so far should have given the doctor an idea of the most likely cause of her pain, and the question chosen to explore the problem should now be a closed question targeted at verifying the diagnosis and excluding sinister causes. The doctor uses their understanding of the probability of diseases based on prevalence, showing a willingness to accept uncertainty but with a strong and reasonable knowledge of effective examination and safety netting. The doctor should also demonstrate an ability to share this risk with the patient.

> ### Positive CSA indicators
> - Uses an incremental approach, using time and accepting uncertainty.
> - Gathers information from history taking, examination and investigation in a systematic and efficient manner.
> - Is appropriately selective in the choice of enquiries, examinations and investigation.

Doctor: *"I would like to ask you some specific questions to get a better understanding of the problem." (signposting).*

The doctor screens for radicular pains, sphincter function, systemic changes, etc., depending on their suspicions and excludes any red flags. Checks for drug history, etc.

Examination: normal neurology lower limb. Non-specific low back pain. No spinous process tenderness. Good range of truncal movement. Normal SLR.

> ### Negative CSA indicators
> - Uses a rigid approach to consulting that fails to be sufficiently responsive to the patient's contribution.
> - Is disorganised/unsystematic in gathering information.
> - Data gathering does not appear to be guided by the probabilities of disease.

Chapter 16

Undifferentiated problems and dealing with uncertainty

Sometimes patients present with symptoms that are diagnostically challenging, requiring some acceptance of uncertainty by the doctor. It is easier to deal with these challenges when the patient is encouraged to participate in the decision-making. Dealing with problems which do not have a clear diagnostic feature is a very good example of one of the benefits of patient-centredness, as the doctor is still able to understand the patient's experience of the problem despite the difficulties of making a definitive diagnosis. They can use their knowledge of likelihoods based on prevalence to recognise the possible causes while simultaneously excluding the signs of sinister alternative causes.

The doctor is still able to understand the patient's perspective of the situation and address the patient's concerns using their broad knowledge of common presentations, but will have to safety net appropriately to reflect their understanding of the principles of working/dealing with uncertain diagnosis. The patient is likely to understand the doctor's views and thoughts if these views are shared openly, and also the patient's perspectives to achieve a shared understanding. The explanation should be given in a way to show the doctor's responsiveness to the patient's preferences. Although the diagnosis remains unclear, the patient (having been involved in the mutual agreement) is more reassured due to the inclusive nature of the doctor's approach. This shared understanding enhances the acceptance of uncertainties and compliance with safety net advice, respecting and empowering the patient's autonomy.

> *Positive CSA indicators*
> - Uses an incremental approach, using time and accepting uncertainty.
> - Data gathering appears to be guided by the probabilities of disease.
> - Works in partnership, finding common ground to develop a shared management plan.
> - Communicates risk effectively to patients.
> - Shows responsiveness to the patient's preferences, feelings and expectations.
> - Enhances patient autonomy.
> - Provides explanations that are relevant and understandable to the patient.

57-year-old man

Patient: *"I want your advice about this mild headache that I've been experiencing for the last 3 weeks."*

The doctor has very little information to go by, so needs to understand the patient's request better. Often patients make a suggestion about the reason for their attending using an opening statement, and the task at this stage is to encourage them to share their thoughts so that the doctor can gain an insight into their reason for attending. The doctor should be thinking about the patient's thoughts and experiences, to try to understand the person rather than simply the clinical problem. Patients have different thoughts and feelings about their problems, and the advice given to the patient should reflect that difference. The doctor should not distract the patient from their train of thought at this stage, but should concentrate on understanding what might be going on in their minds. Gaining insight into understanding will improve the doctor's choice of line of enquiry and often reflects a genuine willingness to develop a relationship with the patient, one that is open enough for the doctor to be able to work in partnership with the patient.

> *Positive CSA indicators*
> - Encourages the patient to participate in the consultation.
> - Explores the patient's agenda, health beliefs and preferences.

Doctor: *"What has happened exactly?"*

The doctor uses an open question to explore both the problem and the patient. The patient gives an account of the problem from their experience of it, and this context provides an opportunity for the doctor to gain some insight into the patient's unique understanding of their experience of the problem. This is achieved through actively listening to the patient to understand the patient's line of thought and using that understanding to select questions that are likely to encourage the patient to share their views without appearing illogical and non-structured. Understanding the views of the patient will help the doctor focus the consultation, and prepare for the negotiation using the patient's understanding so as to find common ground for mutual agreement.

> *Positive CSA indicators*
> - Works in partnership, finding common ground to develop a shared management plan.
> - Appears alert to verbal and non-verbal cues.

Patient: *"I really don't understand it; I've felt a little fuzzy in this part of my head – just above the left ear – for over 3 weeks now. I won't really call it a headache. It's really a very mild feeling and not something I can't live with. I've been to the optician, but he said my eye check wasn't due for another 2 months. I've suffered a stiff neck over the last 12 months, and am currently seeing a physio for it. I'm not really sure if this fuzziness would be as a result of these problems I'm having in the neck area, but I have also been a pilot all my life, although now retired. I'm used to my ear blocking and popping but never had any feelings like this before. I thought I'd get your advice."*

Open question gives the patient more opportunity to share their thoughts, and within that context the doctor uses reflective questions to build a wider picture of the patient's experience and perspective. This is even more important in presentations that are easily identifiable and may require some acceptance of uncertainty of diagnosis, as the value of making sure the patient understands any explanation given or treatment offered is more noticeable. Making an immediate assumption of the reasons for a patient's attendance is a negative indicator, and here the doctor has focused on understanding the patient's experience using an open question aimed at exploring both the clinical condition and the patient's experience.

> **Negative CSA indicator**
> - Makes immediate assumptions about the problem.

Doctor: *"It sounds like you've been deliberating on the possible causes of the problem."*

Reflective questions are useful in exploring the patient's feelings about their problem. They also confirm to the patient that their thoughts and feelings were heard. The doctor appears to be focusing on developing an understanding of the patient's experience, and is likely to gain some insight into the nature of the problem the patient has attended with and the context of the problem.

> **Positive CSA indicators**
> - Encourages the patient to participate in the consultation.
> - Explores the patient's agenda, health beliefs and preferences.

Patient: *"Yes. I really didn't think it was anything serious, as I haven't felt at all unwell in myself. I haven't felt sick or experienced any changes in my vision, etc. I had a stent in my heart 6 years ago after my heart attack, so when things like this happen, your mind starts to wonder about things like a blocked vessel. My blood pressure was normal this morning at home because I keep a very close eye on it, and I take an aspirin regularly every day. I've rubbed my hands on the scalp around the area, but can't feel anything. It hasn't woken me up at night or stopped me from doing things, but it's just that I've never been someone who ever gets a headache. I spend a lot of time reading on the computer screen, which the physiotherapist has warned me to stop doing as it affects the stiffness of my neck. I did think it was my eyesight that needed checking but since the optician said my eye check wasn't due, I thought I'd come and see you. I've also recently started using a particular menthol sweet, but I'm sure it can't be anything to do with that."*

Patients respond better in the consultation when they perceive that the doctor is genuinely interested in their contribution and their condition. Reflective questions explore the patient's experience and also reassure the patient that their views are being heard. Formulaic questions are unlikely to give the same outcome, as a question like "What do you think has caused the headache?" may be responded to by "I don't know, you're the doctor", especially when no rapport has been built up. A doctor who is able to approach the patient's problems in this way is more likely to efficiently gain a holistic understanding of their patients.

> **Positive CSA indicators**
> - Explores the patient's agenda, health beliefs and preferences.
> - Appears alert to verbal and non-verbal cues.

Doctor: *"Would you be able to describe the feeling exactly?"*

Patient: *"It's hard to describe, but it feels a little like you would feel at a high altitude, as if you would need to pop your ears, but it's not painful or anything. It's just there, a bit of a nuisance."*

Doctor: *"I can see it has been a bit of a puzzle for you. I'm going to ask you some specific questions to help me understand the problem a bit better." (signposting).*

The doctor uses closed questions to characterise the symptoms more using selective questions targeted at likely causes based on prevalence, to exclude significant sinister causes. Excludes hearing loss and tinnitus, clarifies drug history, relevant PMH, smoking, etc. The approach at this stage of the doctor's experience is to use probability based on prevalence to guide them to choose closed questions necessary to clarify the patient's thoughts and the doctor's agenda (which is keeping the patient safe or making a diagnosis). A broad exhaustive approach will appear non-structured and time-inefficient.

Positive CSA indicators
- Uses an incremental approach, using time and accepting uncertainty.
- Gathers information from history taking, examination and investigation in a systematic and efficient manner.
- Is appropriately selective in the choice of enquiries, examinations and investigations.

Negative CSA indicators
- Is disorganised/unsystematic in gathering information.
- Data gathering does not appear to be guided by the probabilities of disease.

Doctor: *"Is it OK if I have a look at the muscles of the face and check your eyes, and have a look into the eye to see if I can understand the possible cause of the problem?"*

Examination: normal scalp. Normal eye movement and no cerebellar signs. Normal neurology central. BP 120/70 mmHg. Left ear blocked with wax.

Positive CSA indicators
- Is appropriately selective in the choice of enquiries, examinations and investigations.
- Gathers information from history taking, examination and investigation in a systematic and efficient manner.

Doctor: *"I've had a look. There are no signs suggesting that you have a blocked vessel – normally if there is a blocked vessel it would show on the muscles of the face or limbs but they all move and feel OK. The area feels normal, as you observed. Your blood pressure is OK. The nerves in your face and limbs are all fine. There are no signs suggesting a particular cause, and nothing to suggest anything serious is causing the feeling. Your left ear has lots of wax in it blocking the passage, although I wouldn't normally expect this to cause the feelings that you've had. I really can't see any medical reasons why the sweets would be causing the feelings you're experiencing. I'm not sure how you feel about it now."*

The doctor shares his thoughts about the findings and the diagnosis, showing responsiveness to their understanding of the patient's thoughts about the situation. It is important to observe how the explanation offered reflects the doctor's understanding of the patient as a whole rather than simply giving a medical diagnosis using non-jargon. This is a common misunderstanding and a common reason for failure in the CSA, as doctors fail to understand that the stage of explanation of diagnosis is usually the first opportunity presented during the consultation when the doctor will be required to demonstrate their understanding of the patient and the problem. A doctor who approaches the consultation by focusing on the problem and then at some point seeking to discover ICE may not achieve the same level of understanding of the patient's experience, because the questions they may ask could be too narrow.

> **Positive CSA indicators**
> - Shows responsiveness to the patient's preferences, feelings and expectations.
> - Enhances patient autonomy.
> - Provides explanations that are relevant and understandable to the patient.

Patient: *"I couldn't work out what the problem could be either, but I feel so relieved that there's no suggestion of a blocked vessel in the brain, because it has been playing on my mind. Now that you've mentioned this, I do sometimes get a lot of wax in that ear, which can make my ears feel a little full and blocked. I wonder if that might not be helping, perhaps I could get them cleaned."*

Patient's contribution. Patient should be empowered to participate in the decision-making.

It is important to understand that when consultations are approached in an open manner it is likely that the patient will continue to contribute to the consultation throughout the stages of the encounter. The doctor's agenda is to use their knowledge of prevalence and likelihood to exclude significant alternative causes and use red flags and safety nets to demonstrate an understanding of the management of foreseeable uncertainties using these skills. Exhaustive questioning in the CSA which is not guided by the knowledge of likelihood is considered to be disorganised and unstructured, because it is likely to appear illogical and to lack focus and direction.

> **Negative CSA indicators**
> - Is disorganised/unsystematic in gathering information.
> - Data gathering does not appear to be guided by the probabilities of disease.

Doctor: *"It may well be a good idea to clear the left ear of the wax in the meantime and see if that helps the feeling, and we can review the situation in about a week to see if all is well."*

Using time as a tool. The doctor is suggestive in his offer of an option using his knowledge of the natural course of conditions, thinking flexibly around the problem to find a practical, reasonable, logical solution using his understanding of the problem in the context of that individual patient, but keeping the consultation safe using their knowledge of dealing with uncertainties.

> **Positive CSA indicators**
> - Uses an incremental approach, using time and accepting uncertainty.
> - Works in partnership, finding common ground to develop a shared management plan.
> - Enhances patient autonomy.

Patient: *"That sounds perfectly reasonable. I will definitely get the wax cleaned out."*

Mutual agreement.

Doctor: *"I know we're not completely sure of the cause of the feeling at this stage, but you must let me know if anything changes. If you notice any headaches, or feel unwell, you can let me know beforehand otherwise we'll see what the area feels like after the cleaning. It may perhaps be a good idea to hold off the sweets for a while. Although they are less likely to be* *a cause, the problem does seem to have appeared at the same time you started using the sweets. How would you feel about this?"*

Safety net is vital in dealing with uncertainty, especially when time is used as a tool. The doctor should reflect their approach with the use of probability at this stage to safeguard the patient and put plans in place to reflect their understanding of uncertainties. This information goes further to reassure the patient and address their concerns. It is important to understand that the safety net is a crucial part of consulting in a focused manner, as this is an opportunity to respond not only to the patient's concerns but also to the doctor's tolerance of uncertainties.

Positive CSA indicator
- Shows responsiveness to the patient's preferences, feelings and expectations.

Patient: *"I was thinking of doing just that for now."*

Mutual agreement.

Chapter 17

The patient's uniqueness

Every patient has a unique experience of their problem, and this should be understood by the doctor in order for them to appreciate the need to develop an insight into the patient's thoughts and feelings about their problem. This uniqueness cannot be replicated by any textbook, but what is certain is that it can be explored. The doctor should focus on learning how to consult with this in the forefront of their mind, improving their data gathering to reflect their understanding of the patient's uniqueness. Achieving this early in the consultation focuses the rest of the consultation on the specific tasks the patient has presented and more time can be spent on dealing with the main issues and priorities, thus providing the basis on which the doctor is able to build a relationship aimed at achieving a shared decision. The explanation and management stages of the consultation provide an opportunity for the doctor to respond to that understanding of the uniqueness of the patient which they should have discovered in the data gathering stages. Two patients with exactly the same levels of cholesterol may have completely different views about many things, including how they would prefer to proceed with reducing their cholesterol levels, what they are able to tolerate, how they perceive health issues, what their understanding of cholesterol is, their health beliefs, how their life experiences have shaped their health beliefs, how they view their lifestyles, and even how much they are willing to participate in the decision regarding the treatment. An approach to the consultation with the focus on the problem rather than the patient will not achieve this task, and is very likely to be disjointed and inefficient without developing a partnership relationship with the patient.[1]

45-year-old man

Patient: *"I've been feeling numb in both hands for the last 3 months. It usually comes on at night, and gets better when I flick my hands in the middle of the night. It doesn't bother me during the day, but I thought maybe I should see you to find out what's causing it."*

The CSA assesses how the doctor clarifies the problem and identifies the decision the patient has attended to make, by gathering data to reflect the patient's own experience of the problem. The doctor should not be distracted by thoughts about the diagnosis, because this will affect their ability to actively listen. Patients have different experiences of their problem, but the pattern of the problem through the patient's description helps the doctor to develop a relationship with the patient based on a shared understanding of each other's feelings and thoughts. This presentation will be recognised by most doctors, and the CSA is calibrated to present recognisable common presentations, but the task is to develop a relationship with the patient through gathering data to reflect that understanding, and offering advice and management showing responsiveness to that understanding.

Doctor: *"What do you suspect makes the numbness come on at night?"*

The doctor understands the value of gathering data about the problem using the patient's own experience of the problem. It is through the patient's experience of the problem that the doctor gains an insight into the exact reason for the patient's attendance and the nature of the decision or tasks they have attended to resolve. Questions that focus on the problem only distract the patient from their line of thought and do not show an adequate exploration of the patient's experience. This can sometimes be achieved by only using non-verbal gestures or on some occasions, with experience, 'silence'.

Patient: *"I don't know really. Initially I thought I must have slept on it, but I started using a night splint, which the chemist recommended. It got a lot better but has started happening again. I've even changed the way I lie at night, but it's continued to feel numb on some nights. I thought I'd see you in case it's something to do with a trapped nerve."*

The doctor understands the patient's perspective of the problem. This information does not necessarily have to make any clinical sense to the doctor, but it's valuable to understand the thoughts and feelings of the other party in a partnership. This understanding helps the doctor to build a rapport with the patient, to explain the diagnosis to the patient more effectively using a language that reflects that understanding, and to achieve a shared decision.

Doctor: *"Have you suffered from a trapped nerve before?"*

Verbal cue.

Patient: *"No, but one of my friends was recently operated on after he was diagnosed with a trapped nerve in the neck. When I spoke to him, the description of the pains he was having prior to the operation were different from mine. I'm not experiencing any neck pains like he did. I'm hoping the numbness isn't from the neck, as he hasn't yet recovered and it's been 2 months since his major operation."*

Even though the information does not necessary help the doctor diagnose the cause of the problem, it helps the doctor appreciate why the patient has attended. The doctor is likely to empathise more appropriately without trivialising the patient's presentation. This understanding is important in weighing up the amount of information the doctor would need during the explanation phase of the consultation.

Doctor: *"Sorry to hear about your friend, and I'm glad you came to discuss the problem. I can see you're really keen to discover the exact cause of the problem."*

Empathy increases rapport.

Understanding and clarifying the task ahead enables the doctor to focus on the main task, which in this case is confirming the likely cause and excluding any radicular pains.

Doctor: *"How would you describe the feelings you get in the night?"*

The doctor clarifies the symptoms using the patient's own experience of the problem. Using a patient's own experience to describe a problem puts the problem in the context of that patient. This approach enables the doctor to gain insight into the impact of the problem on the patient. The doctor should be able to formulate the most likely cause of the symptoms by guiding the patient to share their experience of the problem. This is useful for generating functional solutions. The CSA encourages doctors to make a diagnosis in a structured way using problem solving and likelihoods, thinking flexibly around a problem and generating functional solutions. The ability to do this relies on the doctor's understanding of the patient and their unique experience.

Insufficient evidence	Needs further development	Competent	Excellent
From the available evidence, the doctor's performance cannot be placed on a higher point of this developmental scale.	Generates an adequate differential diagnosis based on the information available.	Makes diagnoses in a structured way using a problem-solving method. Uses an understanding of probability based on prevalence, incidence and natural history of illness to aid decision-making. Addresses problems that present early and/or in an undifferentiated way by integrating all the available information to help generate a differential diagnosis. Uses time as a diagnostic tool.	Uses pattern recognition to identify diagnoses quickly, safely and reliably. Remains aware of the limitations of pattern recognition and when to revert to an analytical approach.

Patient: *"When I get into bed, it's normally all OK. In the middle of the night I get woken up by a slight discomfort in both hands, and they feel a little numb. It does help when I change the position of the arm. It also gets better when I flick the hand. It's not really been a problem in the daytime, and I haven't noticed any weakness or anything."*

The description of the problem by the patient can be guided logically in the direction more likely to confirm the doctor's suspicion. The details are also valuable in revealing the effects of the problem on the patient, and their perception of severity. Using an open exploration of the problem in this way helps the doctor to appreciate the severity and impact of the problem on the patient. Sometimes these details may need to be clarified further. A common mistake is when the doctor seeks to ask these questions in a formulaic manner, out of context. For example, a patient presents with an earache and the doctor enquires "How has it affected you at work?". This approach is too closed to encourage a sufficient understanding of the context.

> *Positive CSA indicator*
> - Explores the impact of the illness on the patient's life.
>
> *Negative CSA indicator*
> - Does not inquire sufficiently about the patient's perspective/health understanding.

Doctor: *"It sounds like it must be disrupting your sleep."*

Clarifying the impact. The doctor should use this information to offer management advice to demonstrate their understanding of the problem in the context of the patient.

Patient: *"I still manage to get back to sleep. I wake up quite early for my job as a taxi driver, but I have noticed that I'm getting a bit more tired than usual. It's not the kind of pain I can't cope with, but it just worries you when you're not entirely sure. There is no redness or anything. I was getting a bit uneasy about the prospects of the numbness starting during the day, especially while driving. My livelihood depends on my driving, but thankfully it's not affecting me at all during the day for now."*

> *Positive CSA indicator*
> - Elicits psychological and social information to place the patient's problem in context.

Doctor: *"I can understand how that must make you feel. I'm going to ask you some specific questions to help me understand the problem a bit better."*

Using the patient's own information and description to explore the symptoms they are having puts that problem in the perspective of the patient. This understanding helps the doctor empathise more appropriately. How a condition affects a patient depends on the circumstances of that patient.

The doctor uses closed questions to verify the use of a splint, check for neurological complications, systemic health, weight and drug history, etc.

Doctor: *"I'd like to have a look at the hands, is that OK?"*

Examination: normal wrist. Normal motor and sensory function in both hands. Tinel's and Phalen's negative. Full range of movement of the neck. Pulse 70. Weight 110 kg.

Doctor: *"I've had a look and there are no signs suggesting any trapped nerves in the neck at all. The hands look and work OK now, but you've told me you've only experienced the numbness at night time. It may be related to the position of the wrist, especially when you're asleep, and you've said that the night splints helped. Nerves that go to the hand pass through a small tunnel in the wrist, and I suspect these nerves may be being pushed on at night when the wrist is bent. It's probably why the pain eases when you shake the hand."*

The doctor is explaining the problem in a way to demonstrate an understanding of the patient's experience. The information offered is tailored to the patient to enhance their understanding. The doctor has taken into account what they think about the problem, the decision they have attended to make about the problem and their concerns about the situation.

Insufficient evidence	Needs further development	Competent	Excellent
From the available evidence, the doctor's performance cannot be placed on a higher point of this developmental scale.	Provides explanations that are medically correct but doctor-centred.	Uses the patient's understanding to help improve the explanation offered.	Uses a variety of communication techniques and materials (e.g. written or electronic) to adapt explanations to the needs of the patient.

Positive CSA indicators
- Shows responsiveness to the patient's preferences, feelings and expectations.
- Enhances patient autonomy.
- Provides explanations that are relevant and understandable to the patient.
- Responds to needs and concerns with interest and understanding.

Doctor: *"There are a few things that can be done to help the situation. Usually patients who develop this condition benefit from using night splints to help relieve the numbness at night like you have, hoping that it becomes less frequent or sometimes even resolves without needing any specific treatment. I'm not sure if you've considered trying to use the splint for a little longer to see if that would help?"*

The doctor is using their understanding of the patient to tailor the advice they have given regarding the night splint, recognising the patient's previous thoughts about the use of splints. They are negotiating a review of the patient's previous beliefs about the splint. The patient is more likely to understand the reasoning behind the explanation if that explanation takes into account their views or addresses some of their misunderstandings. This approach empowers patients.

Positive CSA indicators
- Makes plans that reflect the natural history of common problems.
- Offers appropriate and feasible management options.
- Management approaches reflect an appropriate assessment of risk.

Patient: *"Yes, the night splint helped but perhaps I didn't give it a good go as I removed it after a week – I didn't realise I could use it for longer. How long should I use it for?"*

The CSA recommends using an incremental approach to offering management options to patients for common presentations. The option offered by the doctor should demonstrate the doctor's understanding of the patient and the impact of the problem on the patient. The way a doctor offers treatment options can demonstrate how they have understood the patient.

> **Positive CSA indicator**
> - Works in partnership, finding common ground to develop a shared management plan.

Doctor: *"If the night splints help, you can continue using them for about 2 months to see if the problem eases, but let me know if within a month you haven't noticed any improvement."*

The duration of time specified should take into account the doctor's knowledge and experience, but most importantly reflect the doctor's understanding of the patient's experience of the problems and their concerns.

> **Positive CSA indicators**
> - Uses an incremental approach, using time and accepting uncertainty.
> - Manages risk effectively, safety netting appropriately.

Doctor: *"In patients who develop this condition in the wrist, often losing a bit of weight can help to improve the condition. I'm not sure how you feel about that."*

Doctor's agenda. The doctor is suggestive, giving the patient an opportunity to play a role in the decision regarding changes to their own lifestyle without being prescriptive.

> **Positive CSA indicators**
> - Encourages improvement, rehabilitation and, where appropriate, recovery.
> - Encourages the patient to participate in appropriate health promotion and disease prevention strategies.
> - Demonstrates respect for others.

Patient: *"I'm currently working with a personal trainer to lose a bit of weight, so it would be an added bonus if that would help as well."*

Mutual agreement.

Chapter 18

Understanding the patient's preferences

Patients have thoughts about their problems. Their thoughts are a result of their own individual interpretation and understanding of the problem, which can often be based on the impact of the current problem on them or on previous experiences of similar problems. The doctor is expected to build up a holistic view of the patient using the information the patient volunteers, to appreciate the uniqueness of that patient's perspective, regardless of how trivial or common the symptoms they present are. Direct questions related to clarifying the patient's preference are mostly less rewarding when they are approached in a formulaic manner or out of context of the patient's line of thought. It's easy to imagine how a patient would feel if their doctor asked them "What are you hoping to achieve from this consultation?" after they have just described their severe knee pain to the doctor, which started the night before and has caused them to miss attending their son's birthday party. This is the type of approach that patients struggle with in real life, when questions are asked out of context and can easily be misunderstood.

Learning how to encourage the patient's contribution to help them to share their views and experiences using active listening improves the doctor's understanding of the patient as a whole, including their preferences. Without a good understanding of the patient's expectations and preferences, it is unlikely that the doctor will be able to tailor their advice and management to show responsiveness to that understanding.

A patient who requests a referral to see a specialist to deal with their heavy menstrual bleed has indicated a preference which would appear to be the reason for their attendance, but on further reflective exploration, the doctor discovers that they had considered seeing a specialist because they were not aware that contraception can be prescribed by GPs. The patient's health beliefs and ideas have shaped their expectations and preferences in the case, and exploring the patient's views sufficiently would then clarify their preferences. The understanding of the patient's preferences therefore is best inferred from an understanding of their views and thoughts rather than a direct pre-prepared line of enquiry, which is more likely to be too narrow or misunderstood.

45-year-old man

Patient: *"Doctor, I've been on these mirtazapine tablets for over 3 months now for my depression. It's made a huge difference in my life, as I'm now able to enjoy things much more than I did before. I've even managed to join a social club, which I enjoy, and life cannot be any better. I've also completed all the sessions recommended by the therapist I was referred to by one* *of your colleagues. He said I should come back to review the medications after 3 months to discuss what to do next."*

The first task is to understand the reason the patient has attended, through an exploration of their understanding of the situation. These thoughts will give the doctor more insight into their unique experience of the problem. An ability to achieve this clarity early enables the doctor to focus the consultation on the main task the patient has attended to resolve, without making any assumptions from their opening statement. Patients should be given a chance to express those views, even when there are none.

> **Negative CSA indicator**
> * Makes immediate assumptions about the problem.

Doctor: *"It sounds like things are going very well for you. What are your feelings about the tablets?"*

The doctor recognises the importance of establishing the patient's own understanding. From active listening, it's clear the patient is very pleased with the treatment, and has attended to make a decision on the progress of the treatment. That decision requires a partnership for it to be considered as mutually agreed. The doctor explores the patient's understanding in preparation for negotiating the best plan of action. The doctor uses a question focused on openly exploring the patient's viewpoint, providing an opportunity to see the situation in the patient's context. This may reveal the exact nature of the patient's preferences and views.

> **Positive CSA indicator**
> * Clarifies the problem and nature of decision required.

Patient: *"Initially when the doctor recommended the tablets, I was very reluctant to take them because of my husband's previous experience with antidepressants. He explained all of it to me, and I do really feel it was the right decision for me. I originally planned to use the tablets for a short time, but unfortunately something has crept up at home. I have a mould problem which the council is dealing with. They're looking for a new place for me in another area, and I'm not sure really if this would be the best time to stop the medication that has worked so well for me."*

If the consultation was not approached in a way that focuses on the patient's own experience, it's likely that the doctor's awareness of the patient's current situation may have become apparent much later in the consultation. The doctor, by gaining this information, understands the thoughts of the patient regarding the decision they have attended to make. The doctor should take the patient's views into account during the negotiation, guiding the patient using their knowledge rather than instructing. A negative CSA indicator is when a doctor does not inquire sufficiently about the patient's perspective of the problem before the decision-making stages.

Doctor: *"It sounds like you're considering staying on the tablet for a little longer."*

Exploratory using reflective statements. Clarification of preference.

Patient: *"I read up on these tablets. I think it's recommended that people take them for a period of 3–6 months and then consider stopping. I wanted to stop after 3 months before this* *housing problem. I'd really prefer to stay on them for now, but wasn't sure if it was entirely safe to do so. I've received a reassurance from the council that the new flat will be ready by next month, so perhaps I could continue taking them until then."*

It is now clear that the patient had feelings and concerns about the treatment, and discovering this focuses the doctor's further approach in not only using their knowledge of the natural course of disease management but also addressing the patient's concerns directly. If this task was not verified, it is likely that the line of enquiry the doctor will use may not be one that will directly address the reasons for the patient's visit and may appear disjointed.

> **Positive CSA indicators**
> - Explores the patient's agenda, health beliefs and preferences.
> - Appears alert to verbal and non-verbal cues.
> - Clarifies the problem and nature of the decision required.

The doctor uses closed questions to verify the state of the patient's mental health. Verifies the social history. Other medication history, etc. (signposting).

Doctor: *"Is it OK to ask you some specific questions to get an idea of how you feel?"*

Examination: well. PHQ-9=6.

Doctor: *"I'm happy to hear about the council's plans. You're right about the use of antidepressants for 3–6 months, but every patient is different in how long they can be on the treatment, and generally decisions are made on an individual basis. These medications can be used for up to a year if necessary, and there is no serious long-term harm in using them for that long. I do agree with you that it may not be exactly the right time to stop the medication, because of what's going on at home. I'm glad it sounds like there is some hope of things getting better, and think it would be a good idea to continue as you had hoped for the next 2 months. I think that it would be entirely safe to do so, and we can review the decision again when we get to that time."*

The doctor has demonstrated their understanding of the patient's experience of the situation in the language they chose to use in explaining their thoughts to the patient. The doctor's understanding of the patient's preference helped the doctor to focus the data gathering to the task, identify the exact nature of the outcome the patient wants, which in this case is not simply 'continuation of the antidepressant' but verifying that it is safe to do so. The doctor demonstrated further responsiveness to their understanding of the patient by choosing to review the agreed plan within a short period of time, recognising the patient's wish to stay on the treatment for the shortest possible time.

> **Positive CSA indicators**
> - Has a positive attitude when dealing with problems and shows commitment to improvement.
> - Offers appropriate and feasible management options.

Doctor: *"I will go ahead and issue you with a 2 month prescription. I'm hoping things will continue to feel OK for you, but in the meantime you can let me know if you notice any problems with the tablets or your mood changes within this period of time."*

Insufficient evidence	Needs further development	Competent	Excellent
	Arranges definite appointments for follow up regardless of need or the nature of the problem.	Suggests a variety of follow-up arrangements that are safe and appropriate, whilst also enhancing patient autonomy.	Able to challenge unrealistic patient expectations and consulting patterns with regard to follow-up of current and future problems.

Safety nets should not be simply a routine appointment to 'see me if not better' but information providing appropriate safeguards for foreseeable problems and dealing with uncertainties, and mostly importantly showing responsiveness to the patient's concerns and preferences.

Chapter 19

Problem solving using the patient's perspective

One of the unique features of patient-centredness is the ability of the practitioner to generate functional solutions by thinking flexibly around problems.[1] This capability is developed through learning how to understand the patient as a whole and to see the 'lifeworld' of the patient to understand the problem they have presented in that context. The management offered to patients should reflect the doctor's understanding of the patient's context, providing a solution to their problem which is workable within the patient's context. The management should not be generic but should show an understanding of the realistic social and psychological context of the patient. The ability to suggest an intervention that involves changing or adapting a part of the patient's life will depend on the ability of the doctor to elicit these contexts.

> **Positive CSA indicators**
> - Offers appropriate and feasible management options.
> - Elicits psychological and social information to place the patient's problem in context.
> - Works in partnership, finding common ground to develop a shared management plan.

55-year-old woman

Patient: *"I've always suffered pains around both of my big toes. My nails were cut back recently by the podiatrist, and they described them as ingrowing. Over the last few days, my nails have become quite sore again. I noticed a little pus come out of the edge of the left one when I pressed on it. The redness isn't getting any better, so I thought I would come and see you."*

The doctor's main aim at this point is to understand the patient's thoughts about their problem by using a line of enquiry that is likely to encourage the patient to share their views regardless of how robust those views are. The data should be gathered in a way that helps the doctor recognise the nature of the clinical problem but at the same time develops a therapeutic relationship with the patient. The doctor should use open questions or statements which explore not only the clinical problem but also the patient's thoughts about the problem. Even though the problem presented might seem straightforward, the doctor is expected to work in partnership with the patient to find a common ground for decision-making.

Doctor: *"It sounds like this particular episode is different from the pain you've had in the past in the area."*

Discovering the patient's thoughts about the current problem. References to previous experiences are a good way of understanding the patient's views about their current problems and would give the doctor an insight into what the patient has made of the current problem. This relationship building through exploration of the patient's thoughts and views is important regardless of the nature of the clinical problem, as it gives the doctor clarification of the patient's reasons for attending and the nature of the decision to be made.

Positive CSA indicators
- Explores the patient's agenda, health beliefs and preferences.
- Clarifies the problem and nature of decision required.

Insufficient evidence	Needs further development	Competent	Excellent
	Develops a relationship with the patient, which works, but is focused on the problem rather than the patient.	Explores and responds to the patient's agenda, health beliefs and preferences. Elicits psychological and social information to place the patient's problem in context.	Incorporates the patient's perspective and context when negotiating the management plan.

Patient: *"This is the second time it has got this bad, as normally it would flare up and settle down on its own. I try as much as possible to keep the area very clean and wear cotton socks. I've been thinking about the reason why it might be flaring up so often, and I haven't been able to work out any pattern to it. I've started using a particular nail varnish remover over the last year or so, and it feels to me that since then there have been more times when it has flared up quite badly. I've had a look at the contents, and it contains acetone and other things. I'm not sure if it's possible that the varnish remover might be irritating the area as most times I put it on, the area stings and itches. I don't know if it's possible that perhaps with the irritation, it then makes it possible for infection to take hold. This is the second time it's got this bad, to the extent of not resolving itself like it would have done previously."*

Doctor uses a reflective question to explore the patient's views, showing their alertness to verbal cues by actively listening. The problem can now be seen from the perspective of the patient, and the nature of the decision they have attended to make becomes clearer. From this point, the doctor is aware of the nature of enquiries to make to help them resolve the patient's problems rather than if they had assumed the nature of the reason for the visit.

Positive CSA indicators
- Is appropriately selective in the choice of enquiries, examinations and investigations.
- Explores the patient's agenda, health beliefs and preferences.
- Does not make an immediate assumption about the problem.

Doctor: *"How bad does it feel now?"*

The doctor explores the severity of the problem. This is a good way to explore the impact of a problem on the patient. Patients often describe severity using a description of how they feel about the problem and its effect on their life in a way that is more open than an answer to a specific question such as "How does it affect your walking?"

> **Positive CSA indicator**
> - Explores the impact of the illness on the patient's life.

Patient: *"It can really be very painful. I struggle to get any shoes on, especially now that we have to wear safety boots at the supermarket where I work. My boss would be happy for me to wear open-toed shoes, but only if I get a doctor's note."*

The impact is a good way to put a patient's problem in context, and is helpful for the doctor to understand the information required when considering practical solutions to the patient's problems. The doctor understands the patient's experience of the problem and the effects on their day-to-day function.

> **Positive CSA indicator**
> - Elicits psychological and social information to place the patient's problem in context.

Doctor: *"You said the podiatrist has cut the nail back a bit. Did they advise you on what to do if the problem continues?"*

Checking the patient's understanding and preferences using active listening. The doctor is now preparing for the discussion they anticipate, using their understanding of the main reasons the patient has presented. The consultation appears logical as the doctor uses a question that suggests a defined line of thought and outcome rather than a broad exhaustive questioning which is often out of context.

> **Positive CSA indicators**
> - Is appropriately selective in the choice of enquiries, examinations and investigations.
> - Works in partnership, finding common ground to develop a shared management plan.

Patient: *"He said the next stage would be a referral to the hospital to have proper surgery done on the nails, but I really don't want to go down that route unless it's the absolutely last resort. I've lived with this problem for many years, but the only thing that concerns me more now is the frequent flare-ups and the occasional infections."*

Patient's expectations and preference clarified through a logical enquiry into their own experience guided by the doctor's understanding of the reasons for their visit. The doctor should use a line of enquiry that shows an understanding of the task, and not a pre-prepared formulaic line of enquiry. This shows their responsiveness to the uniqueness of the patient.

The doctor uses closed questions to check for symptoms of the condition that can predispose the patient to recurrent infections, and confirms the patient is systemically well. Drug and allergy history.

Doctor: *"Is it OK for me to have a look at the toe for you?"*

Examination: mild paronychia.

Doctor: *"The nail looks slightly infected around the outside edge, as you suspected. The pus you observed is likely to be due to the infection. It's difficult to say for sure why it's been happening more often but it's not uncommon to develop infections in the skin around the nail when they are ingrowing. It may be that the irritation you're experiencing with the* *nail varnish remover is not helping the situation as it may leave the area a little sore and irritated, exposing it to infection even more, as you rightly thought."*

The doctor describes the problem in a way to reflect his understanding of the patient's views and experience. The stage of explanation is an opportunity for the doctor to respond to their understanding of the patient's perspective. This can be either by confirming the patient's view if they are correct or empowering them with views which will improve their understanding. This is not the same as explaining the problem to the patient by simply using non-jargon.

Insufficient evidence	Needs further development	Competent	Excellent
From the available evidence, the doctor's performance cannot be placed on a higher point of this developmental scale.	Provides explanations that are medically correct but doctor-centred.	Uses the patient's understanding to help improve the explanation offered.	Uses a variety of communication techniques and materials (e.g. written or electronic) to adapt explanations to the needs of the patient.

Positive CSA indicators
- Shows responsiveness to the patient's preferences, feelings and expectations.
- Enhances patient autonomy.
- Provides explanations that are relevant and understandable to the patient.

Doctor: *"I know this has affected you at work due to the pain. I think the idea of using an open-toed shoe is very reasonable especially as you get frequent flare-ups. It may be necessary to try taking some antibiotics, especially now that it's beginning to bring out some pus – this often means, as you suspected – that there could an infection."*

Suggestive offer with some information to support the reason for the suggestion.

Patient: *"A course of antibiotics cleared it completely on the occasions before when it has got this bad. I will try not to use that particular varnish remover and see if that makes any difference, and thanks for offering to support me with the open-toed shoes – this is probably more important to me than anything because I'm fairly sure the boots are not helping my situation."*

Insufficient evidence	Needs further development	Competent	Excellent
	Uses a rigid or formulaic approach to achieve the main tasks of the consultation.	Achieves the tasks of the consultation, responding to the preferences of the patient in an efficient manner.	Appropriately uses advanced consultation skills, such as confrontation or catharsis, to achieve better patient outcomes.

Positive CSA indicators
- Shows responsiveness to the patient's preferences, feelings and expectations.
- Offers appropriate and feasible management options.

Doctor: *"Although I know you're not keen on any surgery, I'm not sure how you would prefer to treat the parts of the nail that are continuing to dig into the side of your toe."*

The doctor continues to be suggestive in their offer of possible management options, showing a responsiveness to the patient's preferences. This would enhance a mutual decision-making based on the feelings of the parties involved.

> **Positive CSA indicators**
> - Shows responsiveness to the patient's preferences, feelings and expectations.
> - Enhances patient autonomy.

Insufficient evidence	Needs further development	Competent	Excellent
	Uses appropriate but limited management options without taking into account the preferences of the patient.	Varies management options responsively according to the circumstances, priorities and preferences of those involved.	Provides patient-centred management plans whilst taking account of local and national guidelines in a timely manner.

Patient: *"I'd prefer to treat the infections first, and use the open-toed shoes to see whether that makes things a bit more tolerable. I'll also avoid using that particular varnish remover for now, and hopefully there won't be any need for surgery if I don't have any more problems with the nail."*

Mutual agreement based on an understanding of the patient and not just the problem.

Insufficient evidence	Needs further development	Competent	Excellent
	Communicates management plans but without negotiating with, or involving, the patient.	Works in partnership with the patient, negotiating a mutually acceptable plan that respects the patient's agenda and preference for involvement.	Whenever possible, adopts plans that respect the patient's autonomy. When there is a difference of opinion the patient's autonomy is respected and a positive relationship is maintained.

Doctor: *"That sounds very reasonable, but you must let me know how you get on at work, or if things don't work out as we expect – for instance, if you notice that the redness or pus is worsening or you notice any fevers. We can then review other options available to us to deal with the situation."*

> **Positive CSA indicators**
> - Works in partnership, finding common ground to develop a shared management plan.
> - Communicates risk effectively to patients.
> - Does not allow own views/values to inappropriately influence dialogue.
> - Responds to needs and concerns with interest and understanding.
> - Uses an incremental approach, using time and accepting uncertainty.
> - Manages risk effectively, safety netting appropriately.

Chapter 20

Are hidden agendas the unexplored views of patients?

Patients attend to see doctors to find solutions to their problems. They think about their problems like everyone else does, trying to make sense of the cause and treatment of the problem. They often have their views about the possible causes and on some occasions may have researched these causes and their treatments, or discussed them with family and friends. Although the doctor cannot discover every single view the patient holds, they should give the patient an opportunity to express those views. If this is done inefficiently or out of context, the patient will not feel encouraged to share their views, as they may not necessarily be entirely sure of the value of those views in the consultation. These views are regarded as 'hidden' when the patient does not feel the consultation is open and inclusive enough for them to share those views. This situation is also reflected in the CSA as role players are calibrated to only divulge some information when they feel that the doctor has shown a genuine interest in their problems rather than formulaic pre-prepared questions that are asked out of context.

The case below shows a dialogue where the patient has views that could be easily misunderstood as a hidden agenda if they were unexplored or perhaps discovered late in the consultation, making the consultation appear disjointed and unstructured. These views are more effectively elicited if the doctor uses active listening to encourage the patient's contribution throughout the consultation, building a relationship and rapport with the patient.

63-year-old woman

Patient: *"I've come for my blood pressure check. Last week I saw one of the nurses and she took my blood pressure, which was 160/96 mmHg on two occasions. She said it was high apparently, and booked this appointment to see you. I really don't know why as I feel absolutely fine in myself."*

The doctor should actively listen, especially to the opening statement. This gives a good indication of the direction of the consultation and the likely train of thought of the patient. The doctor should not make any assumptions, but be willing to encourage the patient to share their views freely. The doctor should clarify the reason for the attendance and the task ahead, regardless of how trivial the problem may seem. In this case the patient expresses a feeling of denial. The doctor recognises the consultation might centre around the management of blood pressure, but this can only be clarified by exploring the patient's perspective.

Doctor: *"How do you feel about her advice to attend today?"*

Exploring the patient's understanding. The doctor wants to understand the patient's ideas about the situation in a non-confrontational manner.

> **Positive CSA indicators**
> - Explores the patient's agenda, health beliefs and preferences.
> - Appears alert to verbal and non-verbal cues.

Patient: *"I've had my blood pressure checked over the last 3 years, and it's always been absolutely fine. I explained to the nurse that the blood pressure she recorded doesn't surprise me. I've been very anxious over the last few months, and haven't been sleeping very well. I'm sure this would have affected my blood pressure."*

Patient's thoughts and concerns. Health beliefs.

Doctor: *"Would you like to tell me what's happened?"*

Exploring a verbal cue.

Patient: *"For the last 3 months we've been back and forth from the hospital. My granddaughter was diagnosed with a brain tumour, and she's only 14 years old. It's been a very stressful time for everyone in the family. She is very close to me and I've been with her to all her hospital appointments in London, staying awake most nights. Fortunately, her treatment has worked, and they're planning to discharge her in 4 weeks' time. We got the good news today."*

Patient shared their experience. Doctor gains insight into her 'lifeworld'.

Doctor: *"I'm so sorry to hear about your granddaughter. I can completely understand how you must feel. Have you ever had blood pressure issues before?"*

Empathy. Checking understanding. The doctor is guided by his understanding of the reason for the patient's attendance and the nature of the decision they have attended to make.

> **Positive CSA indicator**
> - Gathers information from history taking, examination and investigation in a systematic and efficient manner.

Patient: *"Not really. The doctor had mentioned the blood pressure was borderline once in the past, about 15 years ago. It resolved itself the second time he checked. I don't take any medicine whatsoever, and I'm not one for tablets at all. I look after myself very well, and eat healthily. The last 3 months has been exceptional really."*

Doctor puts the problem in the context of the patient.

> **Positive CSA indicators**
> - Elicits psychological and social information to place the patient's problem in context.
> - Explores the impact of the illness on the patient's life.

Doctor: *"Do you understand the figures in the blood pressure reading, and why we check them?"*

Checking understanding, in preparation for foreseen conversation during the negotiation, and the doctor is more likely to communicate risks and benefits more effectively if they gain an insight into the patient's understanding. They are able not only to suggest options of management but to educate and empower the patient. An inability to achieve this will prevent the doctor from being able to empower the patient or encourage self-sufficiency.

> **Positive CSA indicator**
> - Works in partnership, finding common ground to develop a shared management plan.

> **Negative CSA indicator**
> - Fails to empower the patient or encourage self-sufficiency.

Patient: *"Not really, but they tell me it's fine whenever they check them in clinic. I know it's important to keep the blood pressure low to avoid a stroke or heart attack."*

Health belief. Finding common ground. This understanding is useful as the doctor needs to understand the level of detail they may have to use when explaining information to the patient to improve their understanding of that explanation.

> **Positive CSA indicator**
> - Provides explanations that are relevant and understandable to the patient.

It would be difficult to negotiate a shared management plan with the patient if the doctor did not explore and understand the patient's thoughts about their blood pressure earlier in the consultation. The doctor gained an understanding of the patient's views early in the consultation, putting the problem in context. The doctor is able to empathise more appropriately. The doctor can now engage with a conversation about management of the blood pressure but is more able to show responsiveness to their understanding of the situation and share risk with the patient sensitively and more effectively. Patients are more likely to accept an option of treatment if they feel their preferences and views were taken into account during the negotiation, and that they played a part in that decision. The details about the patient's understanding of their blood pressure may be wrongly seen as a hidden agenda if the patient is not encouraged to share those views.

Patients or role players will not intentionally hide their thoughts, views or feelings, but the views may become apparent late in the consultation if they are not encouraged to share these views.

Chapter 21

Making decisions using the patient's understanding

The dialogue below demonstrates how the doctor uses the information gathered from exploring the patient's perspective to help them focus their line of enquiry for the rest of the data gathering. Clinical decisions and diagnosis are generally made on the basis of the doctor's recognition of the clinical problem presented by the patient, and using the information elicited from the patient's experience to understand the most likely cause of the clinical problem rather than undertaking an extensive conventional history of the problem, which can be time-inefficient. The most effective way to achieve this outcome is to learn how to use the information gathered from the patient's perspective in both developing a relationship with the patient and also identifying the nature of the clinical problem. Sometimes in the consultation, the information gathered from the patient's perspective can enhance the diagnostic outcome or provide the details required for finding a practical solution to the patient's problem.

42-year-old man

Patient: *"I've had this pain around the muscle of the inside of my left scapula for over 20 years. I've seen several doctors over the years, but nothing has really helped. I know it's something to do with my posture, as I've been working with a chiropractor privately over these years. I really don't know what else to do. I feel it mostly in the evenings after work –it's only a dull ache but won't go away no matter what I do. I've come to see if there are any 'modern' treatments available you could recommend."*

The doctor listens actively to understand the line of thought of the patient. To establish the reason for the patient's attendance, the doctor uses a reflective question to explore the patient's experience and thoughts.

Doctor: *"It sounds like you've really struggled with this problem for a long time. Were there any particular treatments you had in mind?"*

The doctor explores the patient's understanding using a reflective question to help them clarify the patient's reason for attending.

Positive CSA indicators
- Explores the patient's agenda, health beliefs and preferences.
- Appears alert to verbal and non-verbal cues.

Patient: *"I don't really know. I've been thinking about it, but I'm not sure about these injections people talk about. My mother suffers from severe arthritis of her knees, and she recently had a steroid injection, which relieved the pains completely. I really don't know how the steroid injections work, and whether it would be suitable for my pain. It just feels like if something is injected into the muscles, it might just take the problem away for* *good. I know it might sound daft, but I also have an air conditioner fan at work, and for some reason whenever I sit opposite the fan, I get more stiff and painful in the area afterwards. I've also noticed that whenever I see the chiropractor, the pain does ease but I can only afford to see him once in every 3 months due to the cost. I know it's not something serious, as I had a chest CT scan 2 months ago, when I saw the consultant for my asthma. I told him about this pain, and he arranged the scan to make sure there wasn't anything serious."*

The doctor's approach has encouraged the patient to share their thoughts about the reason they have attended, clarified the task and the decisions the patient has attended to make, and their preferences. The patient's expectations are best understood within the context of an understanding of the reason for their attendance.

Doctor: *"Can you tell me a little about the pains?"*

Understanding the problem from the patient's perspective. The doctor understands the reason the patient has attended and is more likely to focus their enquiries better and in a more logical way in an attempt to resolve the patient's request.

> **Positive CSA indicator**
> * Is appropriately selective in the choice of enquiries, examinations and investigations.

Patient: *"The back feels fine in the mornings when I wake up, but towards the end of the day after work it starts getting quite tight and uncomfortable just in the inside of the scapula. It doesn't stop me from working, it's just a nuisance. When the area is tight, it feels uncomfortable to stretch my arms out, and it can be a little difficult to find a comfortable position in bed on the days that it's bad."*

The doctor understands the nature of the problem but within the context of how the patient experiences it. This context helps the doctor understand the impact of the problem on the patient.

Doctor: *"It sounds like it can be quite bad some days."*

Clarifying the impact using a reflective question.

> **Positive CSA indicators**
> * Explores the impact of the illness on the patient's life.
> * Elicits psychological and social information to place the patient's problem in context.

Patient: *"There have been some occasions when I've had to lie down the whole evening due to dull pains, but most often I just take some paracetamol and get on with my day. The most difficult is when I try to lift my children up from the floor, it often catches me by surprise."*

Doctor: *"It must be difficult to have lived with the pain for such a long time."*

Empathy.

Patient: *"It's something that I've already accepted I'm going to have to live with, but I wanted to explore the possibility of trying the steroid injections."*

The impact of the problem and the doctor's understanding of the patient's experience defines the task of the consultation and the doctor can help the patient, using their knowledge of the management of muscular pains to resolve the decision they have attended to make. Due to the approach the doctor has taken, they have not assumed the reason for the patient's attendance.

> **Positive CSA indicators**
> - Clarifies the problem and the nature of the decision required.
> - Does not make any assumptions about the problem/task.

The doctor uses closed questions to clarify the absence of chest symptoms, exclude red flags, i.e. weight changes and medication history. The choice of enquiry should be guided by the doctor's knowledge of probability based on prevalence and has to follow a logical pattern demonstrating an understanding of problem solving rather than an approach that uses extensive questioning of all clinical possibilities without showing any tolerance of uncertainties.

Doctor: *"Is it OK if I examine the area?"*

Diagnosis: medial scapula muscle mild pain and muscle spasm. Normal chest. Normal shoulder and neck movement. No midline spinal tenderness.

Doctor: *"You're right, the pains and stiffness you're experiencing are in the muscle on the inside of the scapula, which explains why you have some relief whenever the chiropractor works on your back. You don't have any pains in the spine itself and your neck moves normally without any pain. I can see why you've had problems with it for such a long time, as the muscles feel like they have knotted up in the area."*

The doctor is explaining their thoughts and the diagnosis by describing the reasons for their conclusion using a justification linked to the patient's experience, in order to improve their understanding of the decision-making.

Insufficient evidence	Needs further development	Competent	Excellent
From the available evidence, the doctor's performance cannot be placed on a higher point of this developmental scale.	Provides explanations that are medically correct but doctor-centred.	Uses the patient's understanding to help improve the explanation offered.	Uses a variety of communication techniques and materials (e.g. written or electronic) to adapt explanations to the needs of the patient.

> **Positive CSA indicators**
> - Shows responsiveness to the patient's preferences, feelings and expectations.
> - Enhances patient autonomy.
> - Provides explanations that are relevant and understandable to the patient.

Doctor: *"It's difficult to say for sure whether the fan at work is affecting the muscles in that area, but it would seem quite sensible to think that perhaps it does, as the pain and stiffness tend to get worse after sitting opposite the fan, but I wonder whether you've thought about your sitting posture at work, and whether in fact this might have more to do with the pains."*

The doctor uses problem solving, demonstrating his understanding of the patient's context, finding practical solutions using that understanding.

Insufficient evidence	Needs further development	Competent	Excellent
From the available evidence, the doctor's performance cannot be placed on a higher point of this developmental scale.	Generates an adequate differential diagnosis based on the information available.	Makes diagnoses in a structured way using a problem-solving method. Uses an understanding of probability based on prevalence, incidence and natural history of illness to aid decision-making. Addresses problems that present early and/or in an undifferentiated way by integrating all the available information to help generate a differential diagnosis. Uses time as a diagnostic tool.	Uses pattern recognition to identify diagnoses quickly, safely and reliably. Remains aware of the limitations of pattern recognition and when to revert to an analytical approach.

Patient: *"It definitely does, because I feel much better when I sit away from the fan, but I can see how my posture might not be helping as when I sit opposite the fan, the chair isn't as good as my own chair."*

Problem solving in partnership.

Doctor: *"You're right when you said steroid injections can be useful in relieving pains in some joint problems, but I'm not sure if it would be useful for the muscle pain you're having. Muscle pains like this are not treated using steroid injections, but there could be other ways we can consider to help the pain. I don't know how you feel about this information."*

Showing responsiveness to the patient's preference.

Patient: *"I didn't know the steroid injection can't be used for muscle pains. I'd be pleased to consider other options."*

Doctor: *"I know you see a chiropractor every 3 months, and you find the sessions very useful. Have you thought about perhaps seeing a physiotherapist to see what they can do to advise you on ways to exercise the muscles in that area, and perhaps give you some guidance about posture at work?"*

The doctor thinks flexibly around the problem to find a feasible solution using his knowledge of the management options. The doctor works in partnership with the patient to find a common ground.

> **Positive CSA indicators**
> - Makes plans that reflect the natural history of common problems.
> - Offers appropriate and feasible management options.

Patient: *"That would be really useful."*

Doctor: *"Do you think there are changes that can be made at work to improve your sitting position for now?"*

Functional solutions. Doctor remains suggestive and uses an incremental approach, varying the management to show responsiveness to the patient involvement. Seeking to find common ground to work in partnership with the patient.

Insufficient evidence	Needs further development	Competent	Excellent
	Communicates management plans but without negotiating with, or involving, the patient.	Works in partnership with the patient, negotiating a mutually acceptable plan that respects the patient's agenda and preference for involvement.	Whenever possible, adopts plans that respect the patient's autonomy. When there is a difference of opinion the patient's autonomy is respected and a positive relationship is maintained.

Positive CSA indicator
- Works in partnership, finding common ground to develop a shared management plan.

Patient: *"I've always felt there wasn't anything really that can be done, as the problem has gone on for too long. I will speak to my manager about this, to see if there is anything. Perhaps I'll get some advice from the physiotherapist first."*

Autonomy and health promotion.

Positive CSA indicators
- Encourages improvement, rehabilitation and, where appropriate, recovery.
- Encourages the patient to participate in appropriate health promotion and disease prevention strategies.

Doctor: *"That sounds very reasonable. Perhaps we could meet again in a month or so, to review how you've got on at work and with the physiotherapist advice, but in the meantime if the pain worsens – especially if you notice any change in its nature or feel your breathing is affected – you must let me know."*

Safety net.

Patient: *"Thanks."*

Chapter 22

Discovering the reason for patient attendance using active listening

Patients share their thoughts with the doctor more readily when they feel at ease in the consultation.[1] Achieving this rapport involves the doctor showing the patient that their feelings and thoughts are valued in the partnership. The reason for the patient's attendance is often not obvious from their opening statements. The clarification often comes through exploration of their perspective of the situation using reflective paraphrases from what the doctor heard them say. The doctor encourages the patient to share their feelings through listening carefully, in order to understand the patient's line of thoughts. This understanding and full attention of the doctor on the patient should start almost as soon as the patient starts speaking, as the doctor should be focused on gaining a general view of the reason for the patient's visit. An effective way to achieve this is to have the thoughts in the doctor's mind as the patient starts telling their story. These questions are related to understanding what might be going on in the mind of the patient regarding the problem they are experiencing. This approach improves the choice of questions the doctor is likely to select to help them explore the patient's understanding and perspective rather than formulaic pre-planned ICE questions – ones that genuinely show willingness to encourage the patient to participate in the consultation. Learning to perform in this way in real patient encounters improves the doctor's fluency and efficiency of using this approach, and helps them develop their own unique way of acquiring this information.

49-year-old woman with Bell's palsy

Patient: *"I've recently been diagnosed with a Bell's palsy, and was discharged from hospital yesterday. I was given a course of steroids, which I'm still taking. Things are improving a little, but I thought I would touch base to let you know."*

Opening statement gives a doctor who listens actively an indication of the line of thought of the patient. Using reflective questions that can encourage the patient to share their innermost thoughts are useful at this stage.

Doctor: *"So how has it all been going on for you?"*

The doctor understands the need to clarify the reason for attending. He uses a reflective question to encourage the patient to share their thoughts. The opportunity will allow the patient to share their innermost feelings with the doctor in a way that will make it clearer what their unique experience has been, and why they may have attended. The exploration is done actively, especially at the beginning of the consultation when the patient's agenda is vague.

> **Positive CSA indicators**
> - Explores the patient's agenda, health beliefs and preferences.
> - Appears alert to verbal and non-verbal cues.

Patient: *"The muscle of the right side was affected but is recovering a little now. I'm able to eat much better, and the right eye isn't watering any more. I'm quite pleased with the progress, but I know from reading that it can take anything from few weeks to a few months before returning to normal, that's if it does. I still struggle a little with the computer screen, as it makes my eye water. I've actually managed to work from home, but I'm worried about coping in the office."*

Verbal cue. The patient feels enabled to share their innermost thoughts due to the approach of the doctor in showing willingness to explore the patient's experience. The reason for attending is becoming clearer.

Doctor: *"I can imagine how difficult it must feel for you. What is the situation at work?"*

Putting the situation in the social context of the patient to understand the reason for attending and the nature of decision the patient has attended to make.

> **Positive CSA indicators**
> - Explores the impact of the illness on the patient's life.
> - Elicits psychological and social information to place the patient's problem in context.

Patient: *"I work in the bank, sharing an office with other girls. They're aware of what's happened and have been very supportive. I've been wondering whether it's better for me to go back to work now, or wait a few more weeks to see how things progress. Working from home feels better, as it's easier to deal with the situation. At the same time I was considering whether it's in fact better to go back early, as staying away for too long might affect my confidence."*

Reason for attending. Patient's thoughts and feelings. Patient's unique experience of the situation. With this approach the doctor is able to understand the patient's visit enough to seek a common ground using his learned understanding, and would be able to show responsiveness to the patient's feelings and preferences or respond to the patient's needs with interest (empathy).

> **Positive CSA indicators**
> - Works in partnership, finding common ground to develop a shared management plan.
> - Shows responsiveness to the patient's preferences, feelings and expectations.
> - Responds to needs and concerns with interest and understanding.

Doctor: *"I can understand why that would have been a difficult decision for you. Do you have any occupational health at work?"*

Checking patient's views and clarifying understanding. Preparing for a common ground in the partnership. The information gathered in this way will help the doctor find a feasible management option that will take into account the unique problems the patient encounters.

> **Positive CSA indicator**
> - Offers appropriate and feasible management options.

Patient: *"I've spoken to them at length, and they advised me to perhaps work from home for a few more days to see how I get on. They were happy for me to go in for a few days to get a feel of how working in the office might be."*

Patient's preference and thoughts. The doctor appreciates the exact nature of the decision to be made. This focuses the rest of the consultation on the task. The rest of the data gathering is likely to reflect selective questions targeted at the task, and a data gathering which is logical and follows a clear line of thinking.

> **Positive CSA indicators**
> - Clarifies the problem and nature of the decision required.
> - Uses an incremental approach, using time and accepting uncertainty.
> - Gathers information from history taking, examination and investigation in a systematic and efficient manner.
> - Is appropriately selective in the choice of enquiries, examinations and investigations.

Doctor: *"What do you think of their advice?"*

Clarifying patient's views. Doctor identifies the main task of the consultation. The data gathering is focused on the task. The doctor is inclusive and shows willingness to continue to invite the patient's contribution to make a decision using their knowledge, but one that will suit the patient's own preference and choices.

Patient: *"I think I'm happy with the suggestions, because it gives me the flexibility I need to cope better for now. They requested that, as long as you're in agreement, I get an official sick certificate stating the arrangement."*

Patient agenda is a term used sometimes to describe the patient's reason for attending, and can be misunderstood as a 'hidden agenda' if unexplored. The exploration should not be done in a formulaic way as this does not create the same level of rapport as it would if the patient were encouraged to participate in the consultation by the doctor's active use of reflective questioning.

> **Negative CSA indicators**
> - Does not inquire sufficiently about the patient's perspective/health understanding.
> - Pays insufficient attention to the patient's verbal and non-verbal communication.

The CSA assess the doctor's ability to **explore** and **respond** to the patient's agenda.[1] Often that agenda may require using active listening to encourage the patient to share their thoughts. Once the task is identified, the doctor should focus on gathering data around the task to help them offer tailored advice to the patient. The patient's problem is put in the right social or psychological context, and this context can only be developed if the patient is encouraged to share their unique experience and thoughts of the situation through the style of questioning.

> **Positive CSA indicator**
> - Shows responsiveness to the patient's preferences, feelings and expectations.

The doctor should work in partnership with the patient to agree a mutually acceptable plan that respects the feelings and thoughts of both parties. The CSA assesses how logical the consultation progress is, with the doctor showing control of the progression of the consultation from discovering the reason for attending, exploring the patient's perspective, explaining and negotiating the management plan. These should be achieved through practice by efficiently integrating the skills required to achieve patient-centredness.

Read the other case dialogues that explore how to respond to the understanding of the patient during the explanation and management stages of the consultation.

Chapter 23

Improving time management using the patient's understanding

The CSA assesses the doctor's ability to resolve the problems the patient has presented with to achieve the task of the consultation in a timely manner, and not what the doctor assumes are the problems.[1] This efficiency is often misunderstood by the doctor as having a fixed structure to work through during the assessment, in order to get everything in on time that is related to managing an individual clinical condition. Looking at the published RCGP 'common reasons for failure', it's clear that this approach causes doctors to behave and consult in a formulaic way, not responding to the uniqueness of the patient and the patient's experience, and the patient as a person not forming the centre of their data gathering. Although they may achieve the task, they may not achieve the task in a way that reflects an understanding of the patient, which is what the CSA assesses. The approach should be to know how to develop a relationship with the patient, to enable the doctor to understand what is important to the patient and use that understanding to advise the patient in a way that would show their responsiveness to the patient's views and preferences, thereby enhancing patient autonomy and empowering them. The three domains are interlinked in their assessment, as a poor performance in interpersonal skills invariably means a possible poor performance in the ability to tailor or share the management, or vice versa.

> **Positive CSA indicators**
> - Offers appropriate and feasible management options.
> - Shows responsiveness to the patient's preferences, feelings and expectations.

To be time efficient in the consultation, there are a few steps that will help the doctor to focus the consultation, achieve the task of the consultation safely and in a timely manner, and also show responsiveness to the uniqueness of the patient's experience of the problem.

1. Learning how to discover the reason for the patient's attendance through exploratory and reflective questioning.

2. Gathering data about the problem through guiding the patient to share their story, including their thoughts and feelings.

3. Clarifying the nature of the decision to be made in the consultation.

4. Using closed questions to confirm your suspicions and exclude red flags.

5. Focusing the history and examination on the main tasks.

6. Responding to your understanding of the problem and the patient when giving explanations.

7. Using an incremental approach to offer treatment that is practical and realistic, demonstrating an understanding of the patient's context.

8. Showing awareness of risk by the use of safety nets to reflect the patient's and doctor's agendas.

The challenge is to learn how to maintain a structure in the consultation without having a rigid design. This is best achieved by dividing the consultation into broad sections as below, maintaining some control over the time spent in each chunk. The data gathered in each sector should be approached flexibly in response to the nature of the clinical problem and the characteristics of the patient's experience. For instance, a patient who presented with a severe sore throat may require more time spent on understanding the clinical problem than using the patient's description of the problem to gain an insight into their thoughts and views, whereas a patient who presents to discuss a request for a referral may require more emphasis on the patient's views and preference to enable the doctor to tailor the advice they offer to be more relevant and understandable to the patient.

The rest of the consultation should then be focused using the doctor's understanding of the clinical problem and the patient's experience, and be selective in the options of management offered to the patient. The ability to show responsiveness to the patient's perspective connects all three domains of the CSA assessment.

See the 'recommended approach' below.

Recommended structure to achieve patient-centredness in the CSA

Stage A:
- Allow the patient to tell their story, or facilitate the process using active listening to understand and recognise the clinical problem through the experience of the patient.
- Explore the patient's understanding, feelings and preferences using reflective questions and active listening to put the problem in context, understanding its impact on the patient within that context.
- Establish rapport using active listening and empathy, gathering information which shows you are preparing common ground for negotiation.
- Clarify the reason for attending, discover the main tasks, recognise the problem and the nature of the decision to be made through its description by the patient.

Aim to achieve fluency in your day-to-day practice. Use flexibility to decide the order of enquiry, responding to the style of the patient and nature of the problem. Summarise or paraphrase to check understanding.

Stage B:
- Use closed questions to focus the history on the problem using the knowledge of probability based on prevalence to clarify the diagnosis, accepting uncertainties and using time as a tool in an incremental manner.
- Exclude red flags to address the agenda of both the patient and doctor.
- Focused examination which is selective enough to address the doctor's and patient's concerns.

Use signposts to move from one section to another.

> **Stage C:**
> - Explain the problem to show responsiveness to the patient's preference, feelings and expectations.

Don't simply use generic non-medical jargon, tailor the explanation to the patient using your understanding of their reason for attending.

> **Stage D:**
> - Discuss possible options, responding to the understanding of the patient's perspective in an incremental order. Safety netting to reflect an understanding of the risks/uncertainties of consulting in a focused way.

Think feasible and relevant, not just all the management steps.

The dialogue below demonstrates how patient-centredness improves time management and focus.

38-year-old woman

Patient: *"Basically doctor, I've had enough of this feeling."*

Doctor: *"What's been happening?"*

Facilitating the patient to 'tell their story' using active listening to recognise the clinical problem through the patient's experience.

Patient: *"I've suffered from panic in the past, and I'm 100% sure this is one of those episodes again. This time last year, I had exactly the same feeling when my work situation changed. It feels like a knot inside the stomach and I'm unable to take deep breaths. This time I've tried everything possible to get it under control but I'm not winning, and with Christmas coming, I don't want to feel this way through the holidays."*

Doctor: *"What makes you feel sure that the way you feel now is related to how you felt in the past?"*

> **Positive CSA indicators**
> - Explores the patient's agenda, health beliefs and preferences.
> - Appears alert to verbal and non-verbal cues.

Patient: *"I know it is because I get the same feeling every time I feel stressed. I work in a jewellery shop, and we've recently lost a very expensive parcel. It started the same afternoon we found out about it. This is the same as I have had in the past, but this time even walking exercises – which normally help me – haven't been helping at all, and I'm not sure if perhaps the thyroid tablets I'm taking may be making it difficult for this particular episode to resolve. I'm struggling to get any sleep, and that makes it even harder as I feel so tired during the day. I just don't know really where to go to from here."*

Patient's unique experience. Nature of problem the patient has presented with.

> **Positive CSA indicator**
> - Clarifies the problem and nature of the decision required.

Doctor: *"It sounds like it's really been quite difficult for you."*

Patient: *"It certainly has. The other day, I must confess, I nearly called the paramedics at night because it was so bad I just couldn't close my eyes to sleep at all, but I wouldn't waste their time because I know for sure it is anxiety related. I don't get any chest pains and have recently had an angiogram done privately and everything came back OK. I have so much going on this season, and just cannot bear the thought of being ill. My business depends on me, and I just have to find a way to get better and strong."*

Impact of the problem.

Doctor: *"Sounds like a busy job."*

Patient: *"It is extremely stressful, but I've always coped with the stresses quite well. I've been with the business as a regional manager for the last 9 years, but it's just at times when something major goes wrong, I go into this panic mode."*

Doctor: *"I know you've found exercises helpful in the past to control the feeling – were you considering any other particular treatments for this episode?"*

Finding a common ground for decision-making.

Patient: *"I spoke to a psychiatrist privately last summer about it all, and he recommended the exercise, which I found extremely useful. He also mentioned going on some treatment that will help the anxiety, but requires taking regular medication every day. I didn't like the sound of taking something regularly, so I didn't go ahead with that plan at the time."*

Doctor: *"Are you considering that option now?"*

Patient: *"I wondered if there was anything else that could be used as a temporary treatment in the short term, just to get me through the difficult Christmas sales period."*

Doctor: *"We can discuss these options, but I wondered whether there was any particular reason why you felt the daily regular treatment wasn't the best for you?"*

Patient: *"I just don't want to even contemplate taking anything that has the potential to cause addiction."*

The doctor understands the nature of the task the patient has attended to resolve, understands the reason for the patient's attendance and the impact of the problem on the patient. The doctor now uses their knowledge of the management of anxiety to use selective closed questions to confirm the diagnosis and exclude red flags such as weight changes, palpitations, thyroid problems.

> **Positive CSA indicators**
> - Gathers information from history taking, examination and investigation in a systematic and efficient manner.
> - Is appropriately selective in the choice of enquiries, examinations and investigations.

Closed questions to verify home situation, PMH, drugs history, alcohol and smoking.

Examination: well. Not depressed. Clinically euthyroid. Pulse 75/min regular. On thyroxine 25 µg, last blood test 1 month ago, TSH normal.

Doctor: *I agree with you that it sounds like the feelings you're getting are related to your anxiety, especially as it started just after the incident at the shop. Your recent blood test shows the thyroid levels are normal so that's unlikely to be the cause of how you're feeling, and on examination I didn't see any signs that would suggest the thyroid was not under control."*

Using understanding of the patient's experience to improve the explanation offered.

> **Positive CSA indicators**
> - Shows responsiveness to the patient's preferences, feelings and expectations.
> - Enhances patient autonomy.
> - Provides explanations that are relevant and understandable to the patient.
> - Recognises presentations of common physical, psychological and social problems.

Doctor: *"With the regular tablets, like the psychiatrist mentioned, the tablets we use these days are very effective in managing anxiety, and don't have any addictive properties. You can easily come off them when you feel it's the right time without any problems, as long as the withdrawal is done gradually. Their effects usually start around 2–3 weeks after starting the treatment, and they're usually well tolerated."*

> **Positive CSA indicator**
> - Communicates risk effectively to patients.

Patient: *"You see, doctor, these episodes only come on about once a year, and usually doesn't last more than a few days so taking something regularly may not be the best option for me, but I'm quite pleased to know that they're not addictive, and certainly a good option to consider next time."*

> **Positive CSA indicator**
> - Enhances patient autonomy.

Doctor: *"There are two options we can explore for short-term treatment. One is called diazepam, and it's a medication that relaxes the whole body. It can be taken for a very short period of time to help with anxiety episodes, especially when they're severe, but they do have addictive properties when used for a longer period of time. Although they're effective, they don't solve the underlying problem like the regular treatment would."*

> **Positive CSA indicators**
> - Offers appropriate and feasible management options.
> - Enhances patient autonomy.

Patient: *"I definitely wouldn't consider any medication with the potential for addiction, even the tiniest amount."*

Doctor: *"The second option is a medication called propranolol. This also can help control the physical symptoms of anxiety but by slowing down the system, reducing the symptoms you experience. They don't solve the underlying problem either, just temporarily control the symptoms. They don't have any addictive properties and are usually well tolerated, but can slow down the pulse rate sometimes, especially if used in higher doses."*

Working in partnership by giving the patient options.

> *Positive CSA indicator*
> - Makes plans that reflect the natural history of common problems.

Patient: *"The second option sounds like perhaps the best option for me right now, but I think I'd like to discuss the option of the regular daily long-term treatment if these episodes continue to happen, especially if they happen more frequently."*

Patient able to play a role in the decision-making.

> *Positive CSA indicators*
> - Works in partnership, finding common ground to develop a shared management plan.
> - Enhances patient autonomy.
> - Provides explanations that are relevant and understandable to the patient.

Doctor: *"I think that is a reasonable choice, especially if you're mostly interested in using a treatment that will be helpful immediately. I will recommend using a very low amount of the propranolol, to be used only when required, but I think it would be a good idea to perhaps consider treating the underlying anxiety if it continues to be a problem to you in the future. It would be very useful for us to meet again in 4 weeks' time to see how you have coped with the tablets and work. I think you should also continue doing the exercises, as this is still very helpful both for your mental health and your physical health. Hopefully things will go OK during the busy season, but if you feel that the anxiety is worsening please do let me know or if you notice that the propranolol is making you feel unwell or your pulse rate slows down too much, say to below 60/min."*

> *Positive CSA indicator*
> - Manages risk effectively, safety netting appropriately.

Patient: *"I will definitely do that, thanks."*

Chapter 24

Patient perspective elicited later in the consultation

The CSA assesses the ability of the doctor to adapt their style of consultation to a variety of patients' styles, recognising their individuality and preferences.[1] This means recognising that some patients may not be willing to share their views early in the consultation, no matter how much the doctor encourages them to do so, although the doctor should always seek to get the patient's views whenever the opportunity arises in the right context. It is appropriate to explore a patient's symptoms first, for instance, if the exploration will provide an opportunity to understand the clinical problem, but is best done in a way that also explores the patient's understanding of the problem. The flexibility within the broad structure of the approach used in this book is both logical and non-disjointed if the doctor is able to vary the approach by responding to the preference and style of the patient whilst maintaining a broad control over the sections. What is more important in the CSA is that the doctor maintains control over the four major progressions in the consultation without having to, for instance, continue to gather the history after the problem has been explained to the patient.

1. Discovering the task which the patient has attended through their perspective.

2. Clarifying the doctor's agenda through recognition and probability.

3. Explanation and offering information.

4. Negotiating a common ground using the information gathered.

Insufficient evidence	Needs further development	Competent	Excellent
	Demonstrates a limited range of data gathering styles and methods.	Demonstrates different styles of data gathering and adapts these to a wide range of patients and situations.	Able to gather information in a wide range of circumstances and across all patient groups (including their family and representatives) in a sensitive, empathetic and ethical manner.

In the case below, the doctor discovers the patient's views much later in the consultation.

37-year-old man

Patient: *"I felt a little dizzy 2 days ago when I woke up. It has since eased almost completely, but I thought I'd see you to find out what it may have been."*

The doctor explores the symptom of dizziness to gain an understanding of the nature of the problem. The doctor recognises that the nature of the problem in this case will determine the focus of the consultation. This is most important in consulting with patients who present with an acute symptom.

Doctor: *"What happened exactly?"*

Reflective question to gain insight into the nature of the problem using the patient's thoughts and description. A closed question here is more likely to focus only on the problem. This approach puts the problem in the context of the patient's experience of it.

Patient: *"I felt a little bit flu-like the day before, went to bed as usual. I woke up to get ready for work, feeling a little strange. It felt like the room was spinning, but I managed to sit back down. I felt a bit sick but wasn't actually sick. It felt really scary, but the whole thing settled back down again quite quickly. I stayed in all day, after calling in sick at work. Although it hasn't happened since that episode, I thought it would be wise to get myself checked before returning to work."*

Patient's experience of the problem. Doctor recognises the pattern of a common presentation from the description. The doctor's agenda will be to clarify the diagnosis later and exclude red flags.

> **Positive CSA indicator**
> - Recognises presentations of common physical, psychological and social problems.

Doctor: *"What sort of job do you do?"*

Opportunistic, and in context.

The doctor understands the circumstances of the event, most especially appreciating the problem from the patient's perspective. The doctor may have an idea what the possible causes are at this stage, but understands the importance of developing an understanding of the patient's interpretation to improve their responsiveness to the patient's perspective of the problem.

Patient: *"I work in an office."*

Doctor: *"Has this ever happened to you before?"*

This exploratory question helps in understanding the patient's thoughts using their previous experience or experience of others. Understanding the patient's views is not just a tick box exercise, but a genuine interest in developing a relationship with the patient that will enable the doctor to work in partnership with the patient.

Patient: *"Not at all, but my father suffers from vertigo a lot."*

Verbal cues. Improves doctor's insight into the patient's experience and understanding of the problem. This information will determine the level of information the doctor will decide is appropriate to share with the patient, based on what they already know.

> **Positive CSA indicators**
> - Explores the patient's agenda, health beliefs and preferences.
> - Appears alert to verbal and non-verbal cues.

Doctor: *"Did you think it sounded like what your father suffers from?"*

Responding to the cue. Improves insight into the patient's perspective of the problem.

Patient: *"I spoke to him afterwards, and he said it sounded exactly the same, although he has suffered from vertigo for so many years. I wasn't sure because the doctor said his vertigo was due to debris in the ear, which changes with his head position. His vertigo can be debilitating, as he's unable to leave the house when it's bad. It got me a bit worried when he said it sounded the same. I had some strawberries the night before, but I didn't find anything on the internet suggesting that there could be a connection. I'm really hoping this episode isn't the same as my dad's."*

Patient's health beliefs and concerns. The doctor was able to gain an insight into the patient's concerns because of their focus on the patient's experience. The patient's knowledge of the causes of vertigo is helpful in determining the level of information the doctor needs to discuss during the management phase.

> *Positive CSA indicator*
> - Clarifies the problem and nature of the decision required.

Doctor: *"It sounds like this is a terrifying thought for you."*

Patient: *"I can't imagine how I would cope with my new job if this is something that will continue to recur, like my dad's. This is a job I've worked for all my life and I really can't afford to lose it."*

Patient's concerns are important as the doctor should be able to show some responsiveness to the information when giving the patient information and during the decision-making. This sensitivity is important in dealing with patients, and can only be understood through learning how to explore the patient's perspective rather than using a formulaic pre-prepared line of enquiry.

> *Positive CSA indicators*
> - Shows responsiveness to the patient's preferences, feelings and expectations.
> - Responds to needs and concerns with interest and understanding.
> - Explores the impact of the illness on the patient's life.
> - Elicits psychological and social information to place the patient's problem in context.

Doctor: *"I'd like to ask you some specific questions and examine you, to help me clarify what may have been the cause."*

PMH, drug history.

The doctor should at this stage recognise the nature of the presentation but requires very specific closed questions to clarify the diagnosis using their knowledge of the common causes and their features. This should be done by using selective questions and examination to confirm the clinical suspicion and exclude sinister signs. Most importantly, however, the doctor should prepare to resolve the patient's concerns and main reason for attending, which is not just to get the problem diagnosed but to confirm whether it's likely to recur. Safety netting should be used to take care of the uncertainties involved in this focused approach.

The information gathered so far has put the problem in the context of the patient's experience and understanding of it. It helps the doctor empathise more appropriately, and focuses the task on clarifying the history using closed questions to diagnose a possible peripheral vertigo, excluding signs of sinister causes. Safety nets play an important role in the negotiation of a management plan by demonstrating the doctor's understanding of the management of uncertainties in general practice, and responding to the patient's concerns. Patients are more reassured when their thoughts and fears are understood and taken into account during decision-making.

Doctor: *"Is it OK if I examine your ears and your eye movements to see if this will give me more idea of what the cause of the problem might have been?"*

Examination: normal eye movement. Negative Dix–Hallpike test. Normal bilateral ears, no cerebellar features. BP 127/80 mmHg, pulse 80 regular.

Diagnosis: likely acute viral labyrinth inflammation.

Doctor: *"The episode sounds very much like a vertigo attack because of the way you described the feeling of unbalance, which started all of a sudden and lasted a few minutes. There are many reasons why someone can develop a vertigo attack, although they are all related to disturbance in the ear that affects the body's balance. The episode you experienced sounds like it might have been caused possibly by a virus that has affected the inside of your ear, disturbing the mechanism that controls the body's balance – it's something we see quite often following a viral illness. This is different from what it sounds like your father has suffered for a few years. Usually when the vertigo is triggered by a virus, I would expect the episode to resolve within days rather than continue to recur. It's reassuring that you haven't had any further episodes, and the fact that it hasn't happened to you previously. I don't think it's likely that the strawberries would cause an episode of vertigo like the one you experienced."*

Using the understanding of the patient's perspective to improve the explanation offered.

Responding to the patient's views explored. It's important to note that this is not simply describing vertigo in a non-jargon way. The doctor uses language which shows he understood the patient and not just the problem.

Patient: *"I'm so relieved."*

Mutually agreed.

Doctor: *"Like I said, I would expect this episode to resolve completely on its own within a few days, especially since it has got a lot better already. You must let me know if you have any further episodes, especially if it's much worse, lasting longer or you notice any headaches or feel unwell in yourself. If you notice that this episode recurs, especially within a few weeks of it settling, then you must come back to see me because we may need to check to make sure there isn't anything else that may be causing it. You should know that although your father suffered quite badly with his vertigo, not all types of vertigo are debilitating enough to stop you from working, and there are things that can be done to help alleviate the problem, even if it is the long-term type of vertigo."*

Using knowledge of the natural course of the illness to safety net.

Safety net should be relevant and demonstrate an understanding of the risks.

> **Positive CSA indicators**
> - Makes plans that reflect the natural history of common problems.
> - Communicates risk effectively to patients.
> - Responds to needs and concerns with interest and understanding.
> - Manages risk effectively, safety netting appropriately.

Patient: *"I will do."*

Doctor: *"I know you're not feeling as bad as you felt before, when it started, but there are tablets that can be used to control the unbalanced feelings and nausea, if you do still feel a little unbalanced in the next few days."*

> **Positive CSA indicators**
> - Offers appropriate and feasible management options.
> - Uses an incremental approach, using time and accepting uncertainty.

Patient: *"I would rather not take anything if I can avoid it, as I really feel OK now."*

Patient empowered to make decisions because the option was offered as a suggestion and not instructed.

> **Positive CSA indicators**
> - Shows responsiveness to the patient's preferences, feelings and expectations.
> - Enhances patient autonomy.

Chapter 25

Health beliefs

The main purpose of patient-centredness is to empower the patient to play an active role where necessary in decisions related to their health.[4] To achieve a mutually agreed decision from the consultation, the doctor has to develop an understanding of how the patient feels and what they prefer. The patient's and doctor's thoughts should be taken into account for a shared decision to be possible. The CSA assesses the ability of the doctor to work in partnership with the patient, using their understanding of the value of shared decisions in empowering the patient to participate in the decision-making.[1] For the doctor to achieve this balance, they need to establish the patient's own health beliefs to help them find a common ground for agreement.

67-year-old man

Patient: *"I've been taking simvastatin for the last 6 years. It's helped my cholesterol level come down a lot, but I'm wondering if you think perhaps I could cut them down now to 10 mg from 20 mg. My last cholesterol was 4.1 and it has been less than 5 since I've been on simvastatin."*

The doctor does not make any assumptions about the task ahead, but clarifies the reasons for the patient's attendance. Using active listening, the doctor explores the line of thought of the patient to develop an understanding of their unique experience and the reason for their request. An assumption would be to consider that the patient had wanted to cut down the tablet because they do not like to take statins, for instance.

Doctor: *"Why have you considered cutting down on the medication?"*

Exploratory and reflective, demonstrating active listening and following a logical approach in context.

Patient: *"It's not that they're causing me any problems. When I started these tablets 5 years ago, I saw one of the nurses for a health check and she mentioned that men like me should be on 20 mg and she increased it from 10 mg to 20 mg. Since then I've been on 20 mg despite my cholesterol being very good every year, but I read the leaflet the other day and it mentioned about skin rashes. I've had these scaly scabs on the top of my head for over a year. I wasn't sure if the medication was anything to do with these rashes – I haven't shown them to any doctor before. Although I thought about cutting the tablets down myself, I wouldn't want to do that unless I'd discussed it with you. I can't remember having the rashes when I was on 10 mg – and I was actually doing quite well on 10 mg."*

Some patients will share their thoughts in their description of the problem. The doctor should pay attention to these thoughts, to gain an understanding of how the patient feels about the situation. The patient's experience clarifies the reason for their attendance.

Doctor: *"Do you understand the cholesterol and the treatments well?"*

The doctor explores the understanding of the patient in preparation for the discussion they have clarified as the patient's main reason for attending. This focus can only be achieved if the patient's perspective is sufficiently understood.

Patient: *"From the little I know, they reduce the risk of heart attacks and stroke. I take them regularly, and have always been careful with my diet and lifestyle. I walk every day, and spend a lot of time in the gym doing cardio exercises."*

Patient's context.

Doctor: *"Did you consider the possibility of the cholesterol level going up if we decide to reduce the dose today?"*

Checking patient's understanding. Finding a common ground for negotiation.

Patient: *"That worried me a lot. I wouldn't really want that to happen, but the levels have been quite normal even when I was on 10 mg. I would really like to monitor assuming we decide to reduce the dose today."*

Patient's preferences and concerns.

The main task is not just to reduce the cholesterol tablet but to determine whether it is safe to do so, and a request for an arrangement to be put in place for the patient to feel reassured. This level of understanding of the reason for a patient's attendance can only be gained efficiently through reflective exploration of the patient's perspective.

The doctor clarifies other aspects of CVD risk management using closed questions. Smoking, exercise, diet and exercise. PMH and other medications. QRISK.

Doctor: *"Is it OK if I have look at the rash and check your blood pressure?"*

Diagnosis: solar keratosis. BP 124/70 mmHg, cholesterol 4.1.

Doctor: *"I've looked at the top of your head. The rash has an appearance similar to those we see on the skin in areas that have been damaged by exposure to the sun for many years. It would be unusual for the cholesterol tablets to cause a rash like this. I think it's sensible to lower the dose of the cholesterol tablets, especially as you've been eating very healthy meals and doing lots of exercises. These will help your cholesterol even further if you continue. The dose of the cholesterol tablets isn't determined only by whether someone is male or female,* *although men usually have a higher risk than women of heart problems, if everything else is the same. We're all different, and the decision about what is suitable for each person is made on an individual basis, and in your case your risk of heart problems or stroke is very low, especially considering your current lifestyle, and I would encourage you to continue. Perhaps we can repeat the cholesterol blood tests in the next 6 to 12 months, to make sure it hasn't gone up."*

The explanation reflects the doctor's understanding of the patient. The doctor uses their explanation to address the patient's health belief and empower them. This is achieved by approaching the consultation from the patient's perspective. Health promotion in context. Follow-up feasible and takes into account the doctor's knowledge of the natural course of the problem, and the patient's perspective.

> *Positive CSA indicators*
> - Shows responsiveness to the patient's preferences, feelings and expectations.
> - Enhances patient autonomy.
> - Provides explanations that are relevant and understandable to the patient.
> - Works in partnership, finding common ground to develop a shared management plan.
> - Makes plans that reflect the natural history of common problems.
> - Offers appropriate and feasible management options.
> - Management approaches reflect an appropriate assessment of risk.

Insufficient evidence	Needs further development	Competent	Excellent
From the available evidence, the doctor's performance cannot be placed on a higher point of this developmental scale.	Provides explanations that are medically correct but doctor-centred.	Uses the patient's understanding to help improve the explanation offered.	Uses a variety of communication techniques and materials (e.g. written or electronic) to adapt explanations to the needs of the patient.

> *Positive CSA indicators*
> - Encourages improvement, rehabilitation and, where appropriate, recovery.
> - Encourages the patient to participate in appropriate health promotion and disease prevention strategies.

Patient: *"Thanks. I will definitely continue working on my exercises and see what the levels are in a year's time."*

Chapter 26

Impact of the problem and the influence on decisions

The impact of the problem on the patient, and how they feel about the problem, can influence the scope of the conversation during the decision-making stages of the consultation, and the range of intervention the doctor may offer to the patient in response to that severity and effect. The doctor should aim to vary the management options offered to the patient to reflect their understanding of that individual patient's experience[1] by giving advice that is relevant and feasible to the patient's experience without affecting the patient's safety. They should do this using their knowledge of the management of common conditions to provide a robust safety net and exclude red flags.[1] The impact of the problem is best appreciated within the context of the patient's description of their own experience of the problem, as narrow questions like "How has the pain affected you at work?" may not yield the same outcome as asking a patient "How bad have your pains been?" The second question is likely to help the doctor understand the severity of the problem and its impact on the patient and others (work, family, etc.) simultaneously.

63-year-old woman

Patient: *"It's about my fidgety legs. I can't seem to control the urge to move them, especially at night in bed. It feels awful – I get some relief when I move, but the feeling returns quite quickly. I've lived with this for almost 15 years. To be honest, it doesn't happen every day and doesn't affect my walking or anything, but I thought I'd talk you to see if there are things I can do to help."*

Active listening involves listening to people in such a way as to understand the direction of their thoughts and the real message they are trying to communicate. This involves careful observation of both verbal and non-verbal cues. This stage of the consultation is the most important and often the most neglected, because the doctor occupies their mind with thoughts of the clinical problem rather than focusing on understanding the patient's reason for attending, especially when the problem is not acute. An assumption of the task at this stage will lead to a disjointed consultation which may not achieve the task the patient has attended to resolve. At this stage it is important to build a relationship with the patient based on a shared understanding of the reason for their visit, without appearing to focus more on achieving the doctor's agenda – which is to recognise the clinical problem and exclude potential alternative causes.

Positive CSA indicators
- Explores the patient's agenda, health beliefs and preferences.
- Appears alert to verbal and non-verbal cues.

Doctor: *"Have you discussed this with any doctor previously?"*

The doctor tries to gain an insight into the patient's understanding from possible previous advice from other doctors. This is a useful way to establish the level of information a patient may have. Often in chronic conditions, the patient gains a lot of understanding from previous consults. The doctor understands the value of establishing the reason why the patient has suddenly decided to present, and this is more effectively elicited by understanding the patient's views and thoughts. The information is useful in finding a common ground for shared decision-making, and working in partnership with the patient.

> **Positive CSA indicator**
> - Works in partnership, finding common ground to develop a shared management plan.

Patient: *"I haven't seen or spoken to anyone about it before. I didn't know whether it was something a doctor could help with. It was only when one of my grandsons was diagnosed with 'restless leg syndrome' that it all started making sense to me. The symptoms he had were exactly the same as mine, but the doctors treating him said the condition is uncommon and that it isn't really inherited. I'm sure it must be the same as his, though."*

The doctor gains more insight into the patient's reason for attending. Understanding their level of knowledge of the condition will guide the doctor in using the right level of language in the discussions. The doctor empathises more appropriately by their understanding of the reason the patient may not have attended with the problem for so many years.

Doctor: *"I can understand why you felt it was similar and why you've decided to discuss it. Do you know whether your grandson was offered any treatment?"*

Checking patient's understanding. Verifying expectations using the doctor's understanding of the reason for the patient's attendance.

Patient: *"That was why I thought I'd come to discuss this with you. The tablets they gave him have stopped his fidgeting legs completely, but I don't know whether someone of my age can be treated with the same type of medicine and whether it would be safe to take them in combination with my other medicines for blood pressure."*

The task of the consultation and the decision needing to be made is clearer. The doctor focuses on gathering data to enable them to help the patient to resolve the main reason for their attendance, but also achieving the doctor's agenda, which is to clarify the diagnosis and exclude other causes. Achieving the above through continuing to encourage contributions from the patient is what the CSA assesses.

> **Positive CSA indicator**
> - Works in partnership, finding common ground to develop a shared management plan.

Doctor: *"Can you describe the feeling in your legs exactly?"*

Using the patient's description to recognise the pattern of a common presentation.

Patient: *"It doesn't happen when I'm up and about in the daytime or when I'm distracted, but usually when I'm resting at night. There isn't any swelling or soreness in my legs anywhere when I touch them or anything, but sometimes it just gets a little edgy, as if you want to* *flick the leg. I get a strong urge to move my legs, and I get a brief respite from that urge when I do move them. It doesn't happen every day or anything, and I can't say exactly what makes it bad on some days. I've got used to it over the years, as I didn't think there was anything that can be done about it. I've always felt it was just one of those things."*

Patient's understanding and thoughts. The doctor recognises the possible cause of the problem using their understanding of likelihood based on prevalence.

> **Positive CSA indicator**
> - Recognises presentations of common physical, psychological and social problems.

Doctor: *"It sounds like the night time must be difficult on days when it's bad."*

Empathy.

Doctor is using a reflective statement to understand the impact and severity of the problem on the patient. Reflective statements reassure the patient that they are being listened to and heard, encouraging them to continue to contribute to the consultation. This improves rapport in the consultation.[4]

Patient: *"You're right – on some nights it feels so frustrating that I'm not able to get into a comfortable position. I know this may sound a bit daft but I have on some occasions put my feet into a bucket of warm water to relieve the feelings. It does make me very tired the next day, but I can usually nap in the daytime as I'm retired now. It does play on your mind a little, not that I'm worrying too much about it because I know if it was anything serious it would have gone really wrong by now. I'm able to ignore the feeling when I'm busy. It doesn't affect me during the day at all. I can drive, cook and do things for myself without any problems."*

Putting the problem in the patient's context. This may involve verifying who lives with the patient, how they cope, who makes the dinner, how they spend the day, etc., but the enquiry is best elicited within the context of the patient's experience of the problem rather than a formulaic narrow line of enquiry like "Does it affect you at work?" This may not allow the patient to share their full experience of the effects of the problem like they have done here.

> **Positive CSA indicators**
> - Explores the impact of the illness on the patient's life.
> - Elicits psychological and social information to place the patient's problem in context.

Doctor: *"I'd like to ask you some specific questions to understand the feeling better."*

Signposting. The doctor uses closed questions to exclude peripheral neuropathies, circulation problems, general health. Drug history. Smoking and alcohol. PMH. Excludes red flags and offers to examine the legs. The range of options the doctor explores here should reflect their knowledge of the probabilities of the diseases based on prevalence.

Doctor: *"Is it OK to have a look at your legs?"*

Examination: no peripheral neuropathy. Palpable bilateral dorsalis pedis pulses. Legs are of normal appearance, not pale.

Doctor: *"I've had a look at your legs, and like you said, there aren't any signs of redness and the legs look and feel normal. It does sound to me that the feeling you're getting may well be the same as your grandson's diagnosis from the description of how it feels to you, and I can't find any other medical evidence on examination to suggest that it could have any other causes. You're right to say this condition is not known to be hereditary, but no one knows for sure what causes it or how it starts off."*

The doctor uses a language that shows their understanding of the problem and the patient's thoughts. Explaining the finding in a way to show responsiveness to that understanding, improving the patient's ideas or consolidating the ideas as in this case. This approach empowers the patient.

Doctor: *"You've lived with this condition for such a long time, and I can understand why you are considering any possible treatment due to the effect it has had on you all this time, but I'm not sure if you're aware of the treatment that was offered to your grandson."*

Finding common ground for mutual agreement. Responding to verbal cue.

Patient: *"I wrote it on a piece of paper and have read through all the side effects too – it's called ropinirole."*

Patient's health beliefs. Encouraging patient contribution at all stages improves the chances of working with the patient as a partner in decision-making so the decision would be mutually agreed and shared.

Doctor: *"I can see you had a recent blood test and all your tests – including iron – are normal. This medication can be used as a trial as there is no way to be sure if it's going to be effective, to see if it reduces how often you experience the urge to move the legs, or whether it resolves the problem like in your grandson's case. They're taken once a day in the evening, and like you said there are possible side effects but none that cause serious problems very often,* *especially if they're used at a low dose. I'll give you a list of things to watch out for once you start taking the tablet and if you notice any of these or feel unwell on them, then let me know and we can review the decision. There are a few other options we can explore, but they are largely of similar effectiveness. I'm not sure how you would like to proceed?"*

Doctor explains the side effects and dosing. The information should be given to the patient to reflect the doctor's understanding of the patient's level of knowledge of the condition, making reference to aspects of the patient's knowledge to enhance their understanding of the explanation offered.

Positive CSA indicators
- Communicates risk effectively to patients.
- Shows responsiveness to the patient's preferences, feelings and expectations.
- Enhances patient autonomy.
- Provides explanations that are relevant and understandable to the patient.
- Manages risk effectively, safety netting appropriately.

Patient: *"I will definitely try anything to see if it helps, even if it's just a small benefit."*

Mutually agreed.

Insufficient evidence	Needs further development	Competent	Excellent
	Uses a rigid or formulaic approach to achieve the main tasks of the consultation.	Achieves the tasks of the consultation, responding to the preferences of the patient in an efficient manner.	Appropriately uses advanced consultation skills, such as confrontation or catharsis, to achieve better patient outcomes.

Positive CSA indicator
- Works in partnership, finding common ground to develop a shared management plan.

Chapter 27

Dealing with discordance and the patient's health beliefs

One of the benefits of patient-centredness is its value in reducing or avoiding discordance in the consultation, especially during the decision-making stages. Occasionally, the outcome of the doctor's clinical findings on examination may not reflect the reported severity of the problem by the patient. This scenario is common in the CSA and in real life and can create real difficulties in knowing how to reassure the patient against their expectations. For instance, on examining a patient who presented with a severe sore throat, the doctor finds a normal tonsil and no evidence of severe infection. The doctor should be able to reassure the patient that there are no signs suggesting a serious infection, but how can this be done without damaging rapport between the doctor and the patient or reducing re-presentation and patient dissatisfaction? This is an area where working in partnership with the patient in finding a common ground that both the doctor and the patient agree on becomes very useful.

The case below explores an example of how to apply patient-centredness to avoid discordance in the consultation.

24-year-old woman

Patient: *"I've had this awful sore throat for over a week now. I've tried several over-the-counter remedies, but it's not going away. I wondered if I could get some antibiotics?"*

Opening statements. Opportunity to explore the line of thought of the patient to help the doctor clarify the reason for the patient's attendance, and the nature of the decision to be made.

Doctor: *"It sounds pretty bad – can you tell me how it all started?"*

Doctor recognises the benefit of getting the details of the clinical problem through the perspective of the patient. This can improve the doctor's insight into the patient's experience, putting the problem in the patient's context. The doctor is also actively listening to characterise the sore throat, to help the doctor recognise the pattern of a common presentation, and determine the most likely cause.

> *Positive CSA indicator*
> • Explores the patient's agenda, health beliefs and preferences.

Patient: *"I've had a sore throat many times in the past, but this one is very different. It feels sore on both sides, and the pain is there all through the day no matter what I do. I'm not one to moan about viruses, but if it was a normal cold, I would have expected the pain to be on one side only and to ease within a few days and not take a whole week. I haven't had any fevers, but to swallow even my own saliva is so painful. I've been off sick for a week, and* *that's unheard of. Some of my colleagues at work have also been off sick because of similar sore throats, and one of them said his sore throat resolved after 24 hours of taking some antibiotics, but he couldn't tell me which one exactly. I suspect all of us at work may have picked up the same bug really, so I thought I would see you to get your opinion."*

Patient's thoughts and health beliefs. Impacts of the problem and their preferences. The understanding helps the doctor understand the patient's reason for attending and the nature of the outcome they would like. This is now not just about diagnosing a sore throat as a virus or bacterial infection, but a clarification of the questions raised by the patient. The doctor's agenda is usually straightforward in a presentation such as this, but what is important is the application of that knowledge to help the patient resolve their own experience of the problem.

> **Positive CSA indicators**
> - Explores the impact of the illness on the patient's life.
> - Elicits psychological and social information to place the patient's problem in context.
> - Works in partnership, finding common ground to develop a shared management plan.

Doctor: *"What have you tried already to help with the soreness?"*

This is a pre-emptive question to prepare the ground for any negotiations of treatment. Exploring the patient's understanding and finding common ground.

Patient: *"I've been dosing myself with paracetamol; it does help but after about 6 hours the soreness comes back."*

Patient's unique experience of the problem and concerns.

Doctor: *"Did you think the antibiotics will perhaps take the pain away completely?"*

Clarifying patient's health beliefs. The CSA assesses how the doctor explores and responds to the patient's problem and their health beliefs. Identifying the main task of the consultation.

Insufficient evidence	Needs further development	Competent	Excellent
	Develops a relationship with the patient, which works, but is focused on the problem rather than the patient.	Explores and responds to the patient's agenda, health beliefs and preferences. Elicits psychological and social information to place the patient's problem in context.	Incorporates the patient's perspective and context when negotiating the management plan.

> **Positive CSA indicator**
> - Explores the patient's agenda, health beliefs and preferences.

Patient: *"I think it should. I know the antibiotics cure the infection which is the cause of the pain, but I'm not the doctor."*

The doctor understands why the patient has attended, and the reason for their request. This information places the request in the right context, and the doctor is able to empathise more appropriately. This understanding will improve the partnership and make any negotiation easier, as the views and thoughts of both parties are likely to be taken into account during the decision-making. This is the meaning of a shared decision.

Doctor: *"How do you feel in yourself now?"*

Severity and impact.

Patient: *"Apart from the pain, I actually feel well in myself."*

> **Positive CSA indicator**
> - Explores the impact of the illness on the patient's life.

The doctor uses a signpost to indicate that they need to ask specific questions to understand and clarify the problem. They use closed questions to verify the presence of systemic symptoms suggesting a bacterial infection. They clarify the past medical history and drug/allergies. Smoking history, etc.

Doctor: *"Is it OK to have a look at your throat to help me decide whether the sore throat is the type that will respond to antibiotics?"*

> **Positive CSA indicator**
> - Shows responsiveness to the patient's preferences, feelings and expectations.

Examination: mild inflammation of throat with no exudates or swelling. Temperature of 36.5°C, chest clear, no cervical lymphadenopathy.

Doctor: *"I know the pains have been quite bad. We can tell from the appearance of the throat if using an antibiotic can help resolve the infection. Your sore throat does not have features that indicate it will respond to antibiotics because there is no pus on the tonsils, as you would expect if they were infected with bugs that respond to antibiotics. I think it's important for you to know that even in sore throats caused by bugs needing antibiotics, the antibiotics do not reduce the soreness itself but only reduce the number of days the person experiences the sore throat. Sore throats don't necessarily have to be on one side only if they're caused by a virus, occasionally it can affect both sides. It's difficult to say what bug your friends had, as these decisions are best made after an examination like the one I've just done on you. I know you've already suffered for a week, but it's worth knowing that these types of sore throat infection caused by a virus can resolve on their own completely. There are things we can do to reduce the pains you're getting. How does that information make you feel now?"*

Addresses health beliefs. Using language which reflects an understanding of the patient. Responding to the patient's agenda and preferences. The doctor achieves the task of the consultation, responding to the preferences of the patient. A common misconception is that responding to a patient's preference is doing what the patient has requested, but in this case that response is shown in the doctor's use of his understanding of the patient to improve the explanation he has offered.

> **Positive CSA indicators**
> - Shows responsiveness to the patient's preferences, feelings and expectations.
> - Enhances patient autonomy.
> - Provides explanations that are relevant and understandable to the patient.

Patient: *"From what you're saying, it's possible that my friend would have had a different bug and really you're right, there isn't any way we can tell. I'm not one for taking antibiotics when they aren't necessary, especially if they won't reduce the soreness, which is what bothers me most."*

Mutual agreement. The common ground here is the shared understanding.

Positive CSA indicators
- Works in partnership, finding common ground to develop a shared management plan.
- Makes plans that reflect the natural history of common problems.
- Offers appropriate and feasible management options.

Doctor: *"It depends on what their doctor found when they examined them. Perhaps we can discuss the options for helping with the soreness."*

Positive attitude. The doctor is suggestive and not instructive.

Positive CSA indicators
- Has a positive attitude when dealing with problems.
- Works in partnership, finding common ground to develop a shared management plan.

Doctor: *"It sounds like the pain comes back quite soon after the paracetamol has worn off. Have you considered perhaps adding a different painkiller in between to help keep the area comfortable for longer?"*

Doctor tailors the advice they have given to reflect their understanding of the patient's experience in finding a practical solution. Offering suggestion to encourage the patient's contribution. Finding common ground.

Positive CSA indicator
- Responds to needs and concerns with interest and understanding.

Patient: *"I wasn't sure I could combine anti-inflammatories with paracetamol in that way."*

Patient's health beliefs. Encouraging patient's contributions.

Positive CSA indicator
- Enhances patient autonomy.

Doctor: *"Perhaps you could consider gargling with some warm salt water, as that can also provide you with some relief in between."*

Doctor seeks practical solutions to the patient's problem in the context of the patient's main concern and the reason for attending.

Insufficient evidence	Needs further development	Competent	Excellent
	Makes decisions by applying rules, plans or protocols.	Thinks flexibly around problems generating functional solutions.	No longer relies on rules or protocols but is able to use and justify discretionary judgement in situations of uncertainty or complexity, for example in patients with multiple problems.

> *Negative CSA indicators*
> - Makes immediate assumptions about the problem.
> - Intervenes rather than using appropriate expectant management.

Patient: *"Sounds like a good idea."*

Mutual agreement.

Doctor: *"Drinking plenty of fluids and taking some rest will help your body fight the virus naturally. I know you've been off work for 2 days already."*

Doctor offers the patient options that are feasible and likely to help their problem. The options are not authoritative but suggestive, giving the patient a choice. Health promotion.

> *Positive CSA indicators*
> - Encourages improvement, rehabilitation and, where appropriate, recovery.
> - Encourages the patient to participate in appropriate health promotion and disease prevention strategies.

Patient: *"Yes, I'll try your suggestions and see how it goes. But what if they don't work?"*

Doctor: *"Normally we would expect a sore throat like this to resolve or at least start getting a lot better on its own within anything from a week to two weeks. I would expect things to begin to ease within a week or so, but if you start having a high temperature or it gets any worse, you can get in touch with me in the meantime."*

> *Positive CSA indicators*
> - Makes plans that reflect the natural history of common problems.
> - Manages risk effectively, safety netting appropriately.

The doctor reassures the patient using their knowledge of the natural course of the illness. Safety net should reflect the doctor's understanding of the patient's concerns and address uncertainties in approaching a consultation in a focused manner.

Patient: *"I will definitely let you know if it gets any worse."*

Chapter 28

The patient's views

The importance of recognising the views patients hold about their problems cannot be over-emphasised.[2] The doctor's task is to apply their learned knowledge to encourage the patient to share those views, and then use that understanding to empower the patient.[1] Sometimes the views the patient holds can facilitate the consultation and give the doctor an insight into which areas to focus on in the consultation, especially in dealing with patients who have a good knowledge of their condition.[1] The patient's views are part of their experience of the problem they have presented to resolve, and may be best explored through an understanding of that experience.

The case below explores an example of a dialogue demonstrating how a patient's views can help the doctor focus the consultation to achieve the tasks of the consultation.

| **43-year-old man** |

Patient: *"I've had fibromyalgia for many years, and saw the rheumatologist yesterday. I mentioned to him about an occasional twinge I get in my right thigh. After having a good look he reassured me that there wasn't anything serious going on, but I'm still not sure what could be causing it. The twinges don't happen very often and aren't really painful but I always try not to assume that every pain I get is as a result of fibromyalgia, so I thought I'd get your opinion."*

The doctor, from active listening, understands the patient has attended to get a second opinion on the cause of the pain. The doctor proceeds to clarify the nature of the pain, by seeking to achieve this understanding through exploring the patient's experience and thoughts about the situation. This will enable the doctor to understand the reason for attendance and the exact nature of the patient's intention.

Doctor: *"It sounds like you suspect there might be a reason for the pain other than the fibromyalgia."*

Clarifying the patient's understanding. This will give the doctor an insight into the exact nature of the request. This willingness to encourage the patient to share their views improves rapport and the patient's understanding when information is given to them by the doctor.

> *Positive CSA indicator*
> * Explores the patient's agenda, health beliefs and preferences.

Patient: *"I don't feel unwell in myself and I do get similar pain from the fibromyalgia, but I've been on these vitamin tablets recently. I wasn't sure whether they could have interfered with my other tablets to cause the aches, as I started feeling this particular twinge since I've been* *on them. I buy them over the counter and they were recommended by the rheumatology consultant on my previous visit. I think they contain vitamin D. I wasn't sure whether I would hold off them for a few weeks, just to see if the pains improve. I had a full blood test last week, and was told my calcium level and everything else were all OK. The reason I thought I'd see you was that I didn't want to just stop them, as in the past I've been advised to stop some of my tablets gradually to avoid problems."*

The doctor understands the reason for attending, and gains insight into the nature of the decision the patient had attended to make. The doctor focuses his enquiry to help the patient resolve their problems and questions. The consultation follows a logical path, and is likely to be structured using signposts to move between the stages. The choice of questions is now more likely to be guided by the doctor's understanding of the task ahead rather than broad, exhaustive, conventional history taking.

Positive CSA indicators
- Gathers information from history taking, examination and investigation in a systematic and efficient manner.
- Clarifies the problem and nature of the decision required.
- Uses an incremental approach, using time and accepting uncertainty.
- Gathers information from history taking, examination and investigation in a systematic and efficient manner.
- Is appropriately selective in the choice of enquiries, examinations and investigations.

Doctor: *"Tell me a little bit about the twinges."*

Patient: *"They only come on every few days or so, and are not there now. I feel the twinge just on the top of my thigh where the muscles are, mostly when I'm resting. It lasts only a few minutes, almost like a cramp. It does go away after I rub it, and it doesn't affect my walking and there hasn't been any swelling. It does feel similar to the occasional twinges that I get from the fibromyalgia. I don't normally get those twinges in the thigh muscles, though, which is why I discussed it with the consultant, but he did say it's very possible that it is a part of the fibromyalgia."*

Clarify the likely cause using the details of the problem as described from the patient's experience of it. Learning to recognise clinical presentations in this way is a very helpful way of building an understanding of the patient and the nature of the problem simultaneously, and improves the doctor's efficiency.

Positive CSA indicators
- Recognises presentations of common physical, psychological and social problems.

The doctor uses signposts to indicate the use of a closed question targeted at excluding neuropathy, complications, systemic health, and the use, timing and dosing of the vitamin tablets. Doctor offers to examine the area of concern.

Doctor: *"Is it OK if I have a look at the thigh and legs?"*

Examination: normal thigh. No hernia. Normal neurology.

Doctor: *"I can't feel any signs to suggest that something else might be causing the twinges. It's possible the feeling is part of the fibromyalgia, especially if the pains are similar. Normally*

I wouldn't expect the vitamin tablets to cause the same kind of twinges, especially as it would seem the twinges are very localised in one particular area. I would have expected a more generalised problem if the tablets were the cause, and your calcium level is normal, like you said. It is a little surprising that the twinges started happening just after you started taking the vitamins, and I do think your idea of coming off the medication for a few weeks is very reasonable. With this tablet, you won't need to gradually stop as it's safe to just stop taking them. Even though they're very unlikely to be the cause, it may be the only way to know for sure if they're having any effects on the area. Leaving the medication for a period of 2 weeks should not cause you any problems whatsoever."

Explaining the problem using the doctor's understanding of the patient. Addressing the patient's health beliefs and responding to their preferences. Using a question to clarify the patient's understanding and seeking an agreement.

Insufficient evidence	Needs further development	Competent	Excellent
	Uses a rigid or formulaic approach to achieve the main tasks of the consultation.	Achieves the tasks of the consultation, responding to the preferences of the patient in an efficient manner.	Appropriately uses advanced consultation skills, such as confrontation or catharsis, to achieve better patient outcomes.

Patient: *"I was hoping you'd say that. I will come off the tablets and see if the twinges continue and let you know."*

Insufficient evidence	Needs further development	Competent	Excellent
	Consults to an acceptable standard but lacks focus and requires longer consulting times.	Consults in an organised and structured way, achieving the main tasks of the consultation in a timely manner.	Consults effectively in a focused manner, moving beyond the essential to take a holistic view of the patient's needs within the time-frame of a normal consultation.

Doctor: *"Please let me know how you get on, perhaps after about 3 weeks. In the meantime, if the pains become more constant or get worse, I'm sure you will notify me before then. I think a telephone consultation would be OK at the end of 3 weeks, for us to decide whether we've taken the right decision."*

Safety nets offered to patient must be 'appropriate' and 'safe'. The appropriateness is a reflection of the doctor's understanding of the individual circumstances of the patient. The safety net is a reflection of the doctor's agenda to keep the patient safe.

Insufficient evidence	Needs further development	Competent	Excellent
	Arranges definite appointments for follow up regardless of need or the nature of the problem.	Suggests a variety of follow-up arrangements that are safe and appropriate, whilst also enhancing patient autonomy.	Able to challenge unrealistic patient expectations and consulting patterns with regard to follow up of current and future problems.

Patient: *"I will let you know."*

Chapter 29

Shared understanding, shared thoughts

The CSA assesses the doctor's ability to tolerate foreseeable uncertainties. One of the expected competences in the CSA is the doctor's ability to use a 'wait and watch approach' where appropriate, tolerating uncertainties using their knowledge of prevalence and likelihood and a robust appropriate safety net. Learning how to use time as a tool is a very important part of patient-centredness, and is more applicable and acceptable by the patient when they are involved in the decision-making.

> **Positive CSA indicator**
> • Uses an incremental approach, using time and accepting uncertainty.

> **65-year-old man**

Patient: *"I've been on blood pressure medication for 2 years, but I haven't had it checked for over 2 years, so I thought I'd get it checked today."*

The doctor explores the reasons for patient attendance, verifies the nature of the request, and understands the patient's viewpoint to gain an insight into the exact task of the consultation without making any assumptions. To achieve partnership, the doctor explores the nature of the patient's request using reflective questions targeted at encouraging the patient to share their views and thoughts.

Doctor: *"Why did you decide perhaps it's time to check the blood pressure?"*

Reflective question to explore patient's understanding and thoughts.

> **Positive CSA indicator**
> • Explores the patient's agenda, health beliefs and preferences.

Patient: *"It all started 2 years ago, when I attended A&E with a chest pain. The cardiology team confirmed my heart was all OK after they checked me over with scans, but my blood pressure was a little high. The cardiologist wrote to my doctor to start me on 1.25 mg Ramipril, but I haven't had time to get it checked as I've moved from one area to another because of my job. My doctor mentioned about reviewing the medicine and arranged a blood test, which was all OK. I've now settled into the area as I'm retired, so this is the right time to get things done properly."*

Every patient is unique, and this is what the CSA is assessing. Doctors are expected to deal with patients in their own individual context and adapt their style to that patient. To achieve this, the doctor acquires information to put the patient's problems or requests in the context of that patient's job, life situation, family, etc.

Doctor: *"It sounds like things are a bit more settled for you, so what are your thoughts about the tablets so far?"*

Clarifying the patient's understanding. Doctor defines the reason for attending through gaining an understanding of the patient's views. Preparing the basis for any negotiations. Exploring the patient's preference and direction of thought. These are often seen as 'hidden agendas' but they are only 'hidden' if they remain unexplored.

Patient: *"I take the tablets every day, and they don't bother me at all. I've always wondered whether my blood pressure was really high enough to need treatment with tablets. I remember the level being around 150/84 while in hospital then, and it's always been up and down the few times it was checked around that time. In fact, I avoid getting it checked in clinic, as I believe it's possible that the level goes up when I do. I worry that I'll just end up getting more and more different tablets if it continues to be checked in clinics rather than at home. I've always wanted to check it myself at home, which is what I've been doing. The problem is that I only have the wrist blood pressure machine and I gather they're not very accurate. I really don't like taking tablets if I can avoid it. My father died from a stroke, and this has always been at the back of my mind, so I would definitely prefer to keep the blood pressure well controlled if it needs to be."*

The reason for attendance is clearer. The nature of the decision to be made is clarified. The patient's views, preferences, and their concerns. The doctor can clarify any part of the patient's experience that raises an issue or concern, but it would not show good active listening if the doctor then goes ahead to ask the patient, after they have shared their thoughts and concerns, 'whether they had any concerns'. It is important to recognise these aspects of the patient's experience as one rather than individual separate entities. What is important is to provide the patient with the space to share their thoughts and experience and, within that context, their views, concerns and expectations should become apparent.

Doctor: *"What sorts of reading do you get at home?"*

Patient: *"It has always been around 130/80 mmHg. Every time my blood pressure has been taken at the clinics or hospital has been an occasion when I was either ill, or rushing about, but I don't really want to come across as giving excuses. I really don't think I should have been started on the tablets in the first place."*

Patient's understanding and health beliefs. Reasons for attending. Nature of the decision to be taken. Although the patient attended for a medication review, it is becoming apparent that they have their own thoughts and feelings about the treatment, and this understanding focuses the approach of the doctor for the rest of the consultation to achieve the task that the patient has attended to resolve.

Doctor: *"I'd like to ask you some specific questions to understand your general health."*

The doctor uses closed questions to clarify the patient's CVD history and FH. Gathers information around the patient's lifestyle, smoking and drug history. Offers to examine the blood pressure. The terms in which questions about patient lifestyle are couched can encourage the patient to share those thoughts in a way that will place the problem in the patient's context. For example, if a patient is asked "Do you do any exercise?", the answer is likely to be a short specific answer which may not reflect the patient's thought about their lifestyle, but a question like "How do you generally keep yourself healthy?" may give the patient an impression of an invitation to share their general view on exercise, diet, etc.

> **Positive CSA indicator**
> - Gathers information from history taking, examination and investigation in a systematic and efficient manner.

Examination: blood pressure 121/70 mmHg. Non-smoker. BMI 24.

Doctor: *"Your blood pressure is normal today. The figure is similar to what you've been getting at home, and I agree with you that it is well controlled. It's difficult to say for sure whether the blood pressure is well controlled because you were taking the tablets, and whether it would still have been normal if you weren't taking the tablets. I agree with you – it's better not to take blood pressure medication if it's not needed. I understand your feelings about occasions when your blood pressure has been raised, possibly because of the circumstances at the time. We really can't say for sure what the situation would have been like if you hadn't been taking medication for the last 2 years."*

The doctor explains the finding, taking into account the patient's views about the situation.

> **Positive CSA indicators**
> - Shows responsiveness to the patient's preferences, feelings and expectations.
> - Enhances patient autonomy.
> - Provides explanations that are relevant and understandable to the patient.

Doctor: *"I know you were concerned about your family history, and at the same time not sure if your blood pressure would remain normal after you stopped the tablets. We have two options. The first option is to hold off the tablets for a fortnight to see how the blood pressure readings are, but this will require regular monitoring – perhaps daily – to make sure the blood pressure doesn't go up. This may either mean coming over to the surgery to use the machine, or doing it yourself at home if it's possible to get a good machine. The second option is to continue as you are as the level of the tablet you're taking is very low, and it hasn't badly affected you. Your blood tests are all OK as well. This would mean that we continue to keep the blood pressure well controlled without any risk of it going up. This would mean you would carry on as you have been, but that we continue to monitor it every 6–12 months as usual."*

Doctor understands the views of the patient and is offering the options based on that understanding. Sharing risk information in a way in which the patient can relate to that information. Involving the patient in the decision-making with guidance.

> **Positive CSA indicators**
> - Makes plans that reflect the natural history of common problems.
> - Offers appropriate and feasible management options.

Patient: *"I would prefer to try without the tablets for a few days and keep an eye on my blood pressure a few times during the day. If I notice the level creeping up, I will restart the medication."*

Doctor: *"That's fine. I'm sure you know that the exercise you're doing will also help keep the blood pressure well under control. Perhaps we can meet again in 3–4 weeks and go over the readings and the outcome, but you must let me know if in the meantime the blood pressure level goes up, especially above 140/80, without the tablets."*

Safety netting using the doctor's understanding of both the problem and the patient.

Chapter 30

Encouraging the patient's contribution to improve explanations

In the CSA, the doctor is expected to demonstrate a willingness to explore the patient's 'lifeworld', and the issues of the patient's health from the patient's perspective.[1] To achieve this, the doctor needs to learn how to encourage the patient to contribute to the consultation, discovering the nature and characteristics of the patient and their unique experiences.[2] The doctor varies their style of acquiring this information throughout the consultation, using opportunities that arise in the right context, especially by looking out for verbal and non-verbal cues. The important thing is to approach the consultation with this task in mind. It is often not enough to just allow a patient to talk, and then proceed by focusing the main data gathering on the clinical problem simply to clarify the diagnosis. The diagnosis should be recognised from a guided description of the problem by the patient through their experience to efficiently gain an understanding of both the problem and the patient's experience of it.[1] The doctor achieves this by actively listening to the patient, and using opportunities within that context to encourage the patient's contribution.[4] The reason for striving to develop this understanding is to be able to involve the patient in the decision-making by improving their understanding of the advice and information that is offered to them.

> **Negative CSA indicators**
> - Data gathering does not appear to be guided by the probabilities of disease.
> - Does not inquire sufficiently about the patient's perspective/health understanding.
> - Pays insufficient attention to the patient's verbal and non-verbal communication.

Have a look at these 'explanations of examination findings' from two doctors. Patient is a 33-year-old woman.

Doctor A: *"I've had a look at your knee. There are no signs to suggest a DVT. The tendons around the back of the knee may have been sprained and could be causing the pains you've experienced, because they felt a little tender when I moved the legs and felt them. This would explain why you experienced pain when you sat down with your legs bent, and why you felt the pain more when going upstairs. The joint itself moves OK, without any sign of arthritis. I couldn't find any evidence of water retention around the knees."*

Doctor B: *"I've had a look at your knee. The tendons at the back of the knee are sprained and this is causing the pain you experienced, but the knee moves and feels normal."*

The difference in the two explanations is due to **doctor A** gaining an insight into the individual patient's experience of the problem, and showing responsiveness to that understanding to improve rapport and empower the patient, making the explanation more relevant and understandable to the patient. This is achieved by actively encouraging the patient to contribute their views throughout the consultation.

Beginning of the encounter

Patient: *"I've noticed this slight pain at the back of my right knee over the last week. It's not there all the time, and it's difficult to say what brings it on, as often it will come on when I'm just sitting. It feels a bit sore when I squeeze the back of my knee. Occasionally it feels tight, particularly when I'm wearing tight trousers, when the crease of the trousers rubs against the area. It doesn't feel swollen and it's not red. It has got better within the last few days, but I still don't know what has caused it and so I thought I'd see you to have a look."*

The doctor explores the problem the patient has presented with, but decides to gain an understanding of the problem through the patient's perspective of the problem. This insight will enable the doctor to put the problem in the right context. Within this context the reason for the patient's attendance will become apparent. These reasons are why patients attend with their problems. Patients want their problems resolved but would also like to understand why the problem has happened in the first place. This process is best conducted in partnership with the patient, to understand the uniqueness of the problem to the patient.

Doctor: *"What happened exactly?"*

Exploratory question aimed at allowing the patient to give an account of the problem from their perspective. The doctor listens actively to gain an insight into the uniqueness of the patient's experience of the problem, and at the same time guides the patient to describe the problem so the doctor can diagnose it. Pendleton's model described the value of the patient's ideas, concerns and expectations,[2] but these components of the patient's experience are often treated as a separate part of the data gathering. These can all be appreciated from the patient's experience of the problem using reflective questioning.

Patient: *"I'm a very keen runner, and run two or three times a week. I don't remember hurting myself at all. The pains have only just started, within the last few days, and for no apparent reason. I don't feel it all the time, but when I bend my knee it feels a little tight, especially when I sit down. I know it could just be a sprain, but I didn't want to continue running in case I cause more damage. I thought the best thing was to get professional advice."*

Verbal cue. Impact of the problem on the patient.

Doctor: *"When you mentioned damage, what did you mean exactly?"*

Reflective questions to gain more insight into the patient's thoughts. This will clarify the nature of the reason for attending and the decision needed to be made.

Patient: *"I take oral contraceptive pills, and I remember a TV programme on them, about water retention. I wasn't too concerned initially as I'd been on the tablets for 2 years, until I noticed these slight aches at the back of my knee. I know I shouldn't Google, but I read that water retention can sometimes lead to a clot. This bothered me a little, especially as my mother had a lot of problems with water retention. When she died, the autopsy report confirmed she died of clots in her lungs. This has played on my mind ever since. I had planned to come and discuss my pills with you, but I got a little concerned when the pains started. I'm not sure if this could be the beginning of a DVT."*

The doctor clarifies the reason for attending, understands the patient's thoughts, appreciates her concern and is more likely to empathise appropriately. This information places the problem in the context of the patient's experience and allows the doctor to focus their enquiry on the main task efficiently.

Doctor: *"It must have been a scary thought, and I can see why it bothered you."*

Empathy.

The doctor focuses the enquiry to exclude risk factors for a DVT, checks the appropriateness of the COCP, excludes red flags. They also offer to examine the knees. It is likely the doctor will clarify the occurrence of fluid retention.

The ability to gather information systematically using questions targeted at the problem is a vital part of time management in the CSA.

Insufficient evidence	Needs further development	Competent	Excellent
	Accumulates information from the patient that is mainly relevant to their problem. Uses existing information in the patient records.	Systematically gathers information, using questions appropriately targeted to the problem without affecting patient safety. Understands the importance of, and makes appropriate use of, existing information about the problem and the patient's context.	Expertly identifies the nature and scope of enquiry needed to investigate the problem, or multiple problems, within a short time-frame. Prioritises problems in a way that enhances patient satisfaction.

Examination: normal knee movement. No signs of DVT or fluid retention. Slight tenderness in the tendon posterior to thigh muscles at point of insertion.

Chapter 31

The patient's context

Clinical management in general practice is the decision-making stage.[2] The partnership built up over the initial stages of the consultation is used to establish the basis of achieving a mutually agreed plan.[1] The doctor achieves an understanding of the patient and the problem in the initial stages to create the right environment to deliberate on the best ways to solve the patient's problems. The doctor guides the discussion using their knowledge, but takes into account their understanding of the patient's views, concerns and preferences in choosing the appropriate line of enquiry and treatment options. A doctor who fails to understand the patient's perspective is unlikely to be able to negotiate effectively.[4] They are likely to offer options that are not feasible, or treatment that the patient may not have preferred.[1] Achieving this requires putting the patient's problem in the context of their experience of it and encouraging the patient's contribution throughout the consultation.

56-year-old woman

Patient: *"I've picked up a chesty cough from my husband who has just finished a course of antibiotics and has got a lot better in himself. I do have a strong chest normally but this time the bug is a very virulent one, I think. It feels like it's more in the throat, but I'm beginning to bring up some phlegm. The last time, I ended up in hospital with pneumonia because of a sore throat that progressed into my chest, otherwise I wouldn't have bothered you now."*

Patient gives an opening statement. Full attention should be paid to this, to gain insight into the direction of thought of the patient. Exploratory questions to explore her views and understand her thoughts about the situation. The patient has indicated what they attended for, but what do they really think and prefer?

Doctor: *"It sounds like you're wondering what would be the best way to treat the cough now?"*

Reflective questioning, the doctor listens and clarifies the reason for attending. This gives the patient a chance to share their thoughts about the situation.

Patient: *"I'm not one for antibiotics when they're not needed but I learnt a bitter lesson from that last time. Although it doesn't feel as bad as it felt the last time, I'm sure I've picked up my husband's bug. Although he is much better, his doctor put him on antibiotics straight away when he saw him. I'm just hoping mine hasn't gone onto my chest, although I would really prefer to start antibiotics early even if it hasn't. I don't want to take any chances this year. I've started taking some paracetamol in the meantime. I know my husband's situation is different as he's only just finished chemotherapy, but I wouldn't want to be ill for two reasons. I don't want to pass it back to him again or become ill when I'm his only support."*

The doctor gains insight into the exact reason for the patient's attendance, appreciates the reason for the request, can empathise with the patient more appropriately, and can put the patient's problem in context. This is achieved through choosing a line of enquiry that encourages the patient to share their thoughts and feelings. Within this context, the doctor understands the patient's ideas, concerns and expectations without using 'formulaic' questions.

The doctor understands the nature of the decision to be made. Uses closed questions to verify the nature of the cough, excludes complications and red flags, smoking history, allergies, etc. The doctor is able to focus the data gathering around the task ahead.

Doctor: *"Is it OK to examine your chest?"*

Examination: temperature 36.5°C, chest clear, throat normal. Patient looks well.

Doctor: *"I've listened to your chest and there is no sign that the infection has moved onto the chest at all. The infection causing your cough is likely to be in the throat, but the throat does not show signs of changes associated with the type of infection likely to enter into the chest. I know you were more concerned about the infection getting worse, if it isn't now, but there are no signs suggesting that this episode will progress. I'm not sure how you feel about that finding."*

Using the patient's understanding to give information, addressing the patient's concerns, seeking common ground.

Patient: *"I'm happy it isn't in the chest, but am not sure about preventing it from getting to the chest."*

Doctor: *"You're right – it's not possible to be entirely sure, but it will not make any difference to how you feel or progress if we started antibiotics now as viruses won't respond to the antibiotics. Assuming this was to progress, there are a few signs that can give us an indication that perhaps we would need to start antibiotics. If for instance you notice any fever, cough worsening, bringing up coloured phlegm, or changes to your breathing, you could ring the surgery and let me know. Perhaps I could give you a prescription today to keep at home, and you could then get it dispensed from the chemist in the event that we needed it."*

Doctor responds to their understanding of the patient, varies the management in line with their understanding but remains safe, taking the patient's views into account in decision-making, seeking common ground with the patient within the limits of good medical care. Provides a safety net using a delayed script.

Doctor: *"How do you feel about that?"*

Patient: *"It would be reassuring to know that I've got something in hand in case it gets worse."*

Doctor: *"Continue drinking plenty of fluids and taking the paracetamol, but make sure you are careful around your husband – as I'm sure you know, viruses can be transmitted from droplets."*

To achieve a shared decision, both parties have to share their thoughts and views for the agreement to be mutual. In the case above, the doctor explained the clinical problem in a way that showed their responsiveness to the patient's own thoughts and feelings about the situation.

Chapter 32

Discovering the decision that the patient has attended to resolve

It is important for the doctor to clarify the reasons for the patient's attendance and discover the exact decision they have attended to make.[1] This does not necessarily mean the symptoms the patient has presented, but the exact thoughts in the mind of the patient that made them decide to attend. These thoughts could be simply as a result of the patient's understanding, their concern or just their own experience of the problem. The doctor should not assume the nature of the reason for their attendance but seek to clarify it by encouraging the patient to share those thoughts.

Positive CSA indicator
- Clarifies the problem and nature of the decision required.

Negative CSA indicator
- Makes immediate assumptions about the problem.

68-year-old man

Patient: *"I was away on holiday last week, and suddenly felt feverish. I noticed some stinging and a bit of blood when I passed urine, and I needed to go a little more often than usual. I was seen by a doctor in Germany who diagnosed a urine infection after a dipstick and gave me a course of antibiotics. It has since cleared up but I thought it would be a good idea to touch base and let you know."*

Doctor actively listens to understand why the patient has attended without assuming this just from the opening statement; this clarification must be sought for the consultation to be focused and efficient. This step is the single most important step in achieving a patient-centred, timely and efficient consultation. This task is more effectively done by encouraging the patient to share their own thoughts and feelings, putting their experience of the problem into the right context through their own description. With active listening, the doctor is able to gain an insight into the reason for their attendance, their thoughts about the problem, their concerns, expectations and preferences, without using formulaic questions which are often asked out of context with no correlation to what the patient has just said. This style of eliciting the patient's perspective not only is effective but helps build a relationship with the patient based on a shared understanding.

Insufficient evidence	Needs further development	Competent	Excellent
	Develops a relationship with the patient, which works, but is focused on the problem rather than the patient.	Explores and responds to the patient's agenda, health beliefs and preferences. Elicits psychological and social information to place the patient's problem in context.	Incorporates the patient's perspective and context when negotiating the management plan.

Doctor: *"Did the doctor tell you what caused the infection or what to do next?"*

Exploring the patient's ideas and thoughts. This question gives the patient an opportunity to share their understanding of the situation so far, perhaps through the information they were given in Germany or possibly what they have made of the situation themselves. It is within these thoughts of the patient that their exact reason for attending becomes clear.

> **Positive CSA indicator**
> • Clarifies the problem and nature of the decision required.

Patient: *"The doctor did mention something about a 'benign tumour of the prostate' which can be a common reason why men develop an infection out of the blue, but he arranged a scan which came back as normal. He still said I should get things checked out when I got back to the UK."*

Patient's understanding, reason for attending clarified.

Doctor: *"Did he suggest any particular line of action?"*

Clarifying the patient's understanding of the situation and thoughts, seeking to encourage the patient's contribution. A logical line of questioning demonstrating an understanding of the need to clarify the patient's preferences. It gives the patient an opportunity to share those views.

> **Positive CSA indicators**
> • Explores the patient's agenda, health beliefs and preferences.
> • Appears alert to verbal and non-verbal cues.

Patient: *"He didn't indicate anything in particular, but I read up about the prostate. I think there is a test that can be done to confirm if there is a problem in the prostate. I learnt a lot about the prostate through my father's illness. He died of prostate cancer and I've always had it at the back of my mind that perhaps one day I may have to go through the same painful experience. I haven't really had any problems with the waterworks until this episode. There has only been one occasion that the doctor found some blood in my urine, but on repeat testing it disappeared. I did wonder if perhaps something may have started back then. It has worried me a bit since, that's why I thought I'd see you this time."*

The doctor gains an understanding of the uniqueness of the problem to the patient. Understanding why he attended, what he is hoping to achieve, and his concerns. The doctor can put the problem in the patient's context, and is able to empathise more appropriately, focusing the rest of the data gathering more effectively on achieving the patient's task/agenda. In this case, you can see how the problem has had more of a psychological impact on the patient, and to discuss that with a question like "How did this affect your life?" may not be an easy question for the patient.

> **Positive CSA indicator**
> - Explores the impact of the illness on the patient's life.

This patient attended to discuss the value of the PSA, with a strong underlying concern for prostate cancer. Recognising this, taking into account their background knowledge, gives the doctor an opportunity to tailor their advice to the patient. The doctor is likely to improve the information they offer the patient using their understanding of the patient.

Doctor: *"I can understand how it must feel to have had this on your mind for a while, and I'm glad you've attended today to discuss this with me."*

Empathy.

Empathy is the capacity to understand or feel what another person is experiencing from within the other being's frame of reference.[8] This is difficult to genuinely achieve without developing an understanding of the patient's experience.

The doctor uses closed questions to clarify the doctor's agenda. History of previous prostate problems, current state, history of alternative explanation of the episode, i.e. penile discharge, red flags and completes drug history, smoking, etc.

> **Positive CSA indicators**
> - Gathers information from history taking, examination and investigation in a systematic and efficient manner.
> - Is appropriately selective in the choice of enquiries, examinations and investigations.

Doctor: *"Is it OK if I examine your abdomen for now and check the urine again?"*

Examination: urinalysis NAD. Planned prostate examination.

Doctor: *"It sounds like the symptoms have resolved. I think you're right to consider further exploration to make sure there aren't any underlying causes of the infection you had in Germany. The urine sample I tested today didn't show any signs of infection, and your tummy feels normal. It sounds like you haven't had any previous problems with passing urine until this episode. That makes it a little less likely that you have anything serious going on, but we can only be surer if we examine the prostate through the back passage. It's possible for someone to have just an episode of infection without having any serious underlying causes, but it's worth checking just to make sure all is well, especially with regards to your family history. I think it would be useful to proceed to check the prostate but I would need to explain a few things about it before we proceed. It's difficult to be sure about the positive urine test you had a few years ago, but I wouldn't have expected you to have developed something sinister for all those years yet continued not to show any symptoms."*

The doctor responds to the concerns of the patient. Recognising the need to focus the explanation using their understanding of the patient in a way to improve the patient's understanding of the explanation offered. The doctor provides information that empowers the patient in resolving the issue they have attended with.

Doctor: *"Are you aware of any tests for prostate?"*

Patient: *"I read on the NHS website about the PSA test in detail, and I remember my dad having several of those. I know they're not very specific, and can be positive even when the prostate is fine. I read that the result of the test and physical examination will help a doctor in making a decision."*

Establishing a patient's understanding when giving information helps the doctor to identify areas of the explanation to focus on, avoiding the possibility of appearing to patronise the patient.

Insufficient evidence	Needs further development	Competent	Excellent
From the available evidence, the doctor's performance cannot be placed on a higher point of this developmental scale.	Provides explanations that are medically correct but doctor-centred.	Uses the patient's understanding to help improve the explanation offered.	Uses a variety of communication techniques and materials (e.g. written or electronic) to adapt explanations to the needs of the patient.

Positive CSA indicators
- Shows responsiveness to the patient's preferences, feelings and expectations.
- Enhances patient autonomy.
- Provides explanations that are relevant and understandable to the patient.

Doctor: *"You're right. The test is very useful in determining the risk of prostate cancer, but has its limitations. Assuming the test comes back normal, it may be that the chances of a prostate cancer being present are low if the examination of the prostate is also normal. There is no way to be sure if all is well if the level comes back high, but I'm not sure – if that were to happen – whether you would be willing to pursue further invasive tests like having a biopsy of the prostate."*

Tailored information based on the patient's knowledge. Giving the patient options. Providing information to help the patient make a decision.

Positive CSA indicators
- Works in partnership, finding common ground to develop a shared management plan.
- Provides explanations that are relevant and understandable to the patient.
- Responds to needs and concerns with interest and understanding.

Patient: *"To be honest, this has bothered me for a long time. I would definitely like to explore the prostate further assuming the test comes back as abnormal. It's better to be safe than sorry."*

Patient's preference.

Doctor: *"It's best to arrange the blood test in the first instance and then examine your prostate physically, as doing it the other way around may interfere with the level of the PSA."*

The doctor uses a language that shows the level of understanding of the patient, and it would be patronising to say something like "level of the chemical" when the patient has already read up on and is familiar with PSA.

> **Positive CSA indicators**
> - Makes plans that reflect the natural history of common problems.
> - Offers appropriate and feasible management options.

Doctor: *"I'll arrange the test for you. There are specific instructions you need to follow before the test, so the results aren't affected. I'll give you a print-out of how to get yourself ready for the test – it contains things like how many days to abstain from intercourse, etc. We should meet again a few days after the test, and I'll examine your prostate then. Hope that's OK by you."*

Follow-up. Seeking agreement.

Patient: *"OK. That will definitely put my mind at rest."*

Chapter 33

Dealing with vague symptoms using patient-centredness

The need to develop a good understanding of the patient is even more useful in dealing with encounters where the patient's symptoms are undifferentiated, vague or at early presentation.[2] This is because the doctor needs to understand the patient's experience more to help them determine the amount and nature of the information they will offer to the patient to improve their understanding of the problem or so the patient understands the doctor's thoughts. There is also a need to find a common ground for both parties to share the risk of the uncertainty more effectively.

74-year-old woman

Patient: *"Doctor, I've had aches under both my armpits in the exact area where the lymph nodes are located, I think! It has felt a bit strange and tight at times for a few weeks. It started feeling that way about 2 months ago, but I've since had a normal mammogram and a normal ultrasound of that area within the last month and a chest X-ray. I was told the breast looks all OK, but I still get the sensation despite all these tests coming back as normal. I'm really not sure what to do."*

The doctor focuses on understanding the reason for the patient's attendance, and the nature of the decision the patient has attended to make, without making any assumptions of the task. The task needs to be clarified for the consultation to be focused on the patient's reason for attending and at the same time the doctor should clarify their own agenda. The doctor should proceed with an open question that will encourage the patient to share their inner feelings, especially when they appear to have an ongoing problem which they would have had discussed with other doctors.

Doctor: *"I'm sure it must be a little frustrating to continue to feel the aches especially since the tests didn't find any causes."*

Reflective question showing active listening. Doctor seeks to clarify the reason for attending by encouraging the patient to share their thoughts about the situation.

> *Positive CSA indicator*
> * Explores the patient's agenda, health beliefs and preferences.

Patient: *"I know the tests have been reassuring so far, but it doesn't stop you from still thinking about what the tests may have missed. The hospital staff have been extremely kind and all the nurses were very supportive, but it continues to play on my mind especially when I feel the twinges."*

Patient's views and concerns. Verbal cues. The doctor gained an insight into the patient's reasoning, which will help them to clarify the task of the consultation.

Doctor: *"It sounds like you're concerned that there might be something the scans may have missed."*

Reflective questions. The doctor explores the patient's thoughts, to gain more insight into the reason for attending and nature of the decision to be made.

Patient: *"You know at my age, it plays on your mind, especially when everyone else around you is dying off. Three of my friends have passed away within the last 6 months, just like that. They all had several scans and it appears that nothing was found as well. I'm nearly 75 and it does play on your mind a bit. I know it's possible I could be imagining the sensations that I feel in that area, but I just want to be entirely sure. I feel more comfortable talking to you in the surgery than at the hospital, so I thought I'd come and discuss it with you."*

Patient's concerns and thoughts, reason for attending.

Doctor: *"I can understand how that must make you feel, especially when you lose close friends in such quick succession. Was there anything in particular that worried you?"*

Checking understanding, clarifying the task ahead and the nature of the decision to be made. The doctor focuses on developing a relationship with the patient because of the nature of the presentation and recent normal test results. This ability to recognise a common problem is important for the doctor to focus the rest of the consultation to achieve the task in partnership with the patient.

Patient: *"I used HRT tablets for over 5 years, but over the last few months the doctor advised me to stop them due to what he described as a 'risk of cancer'. He didn't mention any particular cancers at all, and that made me wonder whether there could have been cancer developing already somewhere, considering the number of years I was taking the medication without knowing anything about the risks. I know this could all be in my mind, but you can understand how it feels when you hear stories in the news about people dying because something was missed on the scans. I wondered if there was a blood test that can test for a hormone or something to check for any possibilities of cancer somewhere that the scan would have missed. It hasn't helped me either that I have a useless architect doing my outbuilding, it has been a nightmare in the last few months, although thankfully things are a lot better now. I can assure you that I'm not depressed or anything."*

Patient's thoughts, concerns and understanding have become clear. The doctor understands the patient's expectation from the encounter and can now focus the consultation more effectively to achieve the task of the consultation.

Insufficient evidence	Needs further development	Competent	Excellent
	Accumulates information from the patient that is mainly relevant to their problem. Uses existing information in the patient records.	Systematically gathers information, using questions appropriately targeted to the problem without affecting patient safety. Understands the importance of, and makes appropriate use of, existing information about the problem and the patient's context.	Expertly identifies the nature and scope of enquiry needed to investigate the problem, or multiple problems, within a short time-frame. Prioritises problems in a way that enhances patient satisfaction.

Positive CSA indicators
- Is appropriately selective in the choice of enquiries, examinations and investigations.
- Gathers information from history taking, examination and investigation in a systematic and efficient manner.

Doctor: *"I can understand why it would have worried you. I'd like to ask you some specific questions to help me understand the situation better."*

The doctor proceeds to clarify the absence of any systemic features of illness, clarifies the nature of the sensation the patient is experiencing, but most important clarifies the situation at home and the ongoing projects and stresses. Drug history. PMH.

The doctor focuses on gathering information helpful in reassuring the patient, especially around the risk from HRT, excludes red flags. The social context of the patient is important with regards to the recent building work going on. This information and context would have only been possible as a result of the doctor encouraging the patient's contributions.

Doctor: *"Is it OK if I have a look at the area?"*

Examination: normal axilla. No lymph node. General examination normal, BP 125/70 mmHg. Chest clear.

Doctor: *"I know you've been very worried, especially about the risk of having used the HRT for over 5 years. You're right about the risk of cancers with HRT, but the risks are really very small, especially when you have stopped using the medication. It's very reassuring that the mammogram came back OK, as we know the breast is the main area at risk. You feel very well in yourself and don't have any specific symptoms that would suggest an underlying problem like cancer, but I know from what you've said that some of your friends also had normal scans before passing away. There aren't really any blood tests that can be used to check or diagnose cancer, and if you had anything like that it would have been likely that you would have some symptoms, such as losing weight. I've seen your recent blood test results, and they are all OK, especially the test which tells us about the blood count. I'm not sure how you feel about this now."*

Giving information in a way that demonstrates an understanding of the patient's unique experience. Achieving the task of the consultation taking into account the patient's perspective. Using the patient's understanding to improve the quality of the information given to the patient to improve their understanding.

Patient: *"I'm glad to hear the risks are low and that you feel there are no signs suggesting a problem."*

Doctor: *"I know you said things are a bit more settled now at home with the building work, but you can let me know any time if you notice or feel anything has changed in any way, if you lose weight or feel unwell in yourself. The most important thing from the breast point of view is to continue to do regular examinations using the instruction leaflet that I will give you, to keep an eye on the area until your next routine mammogram."*

Safety netting should reflect the doctor's understanding of the patient's concerns, any foreseeable uncertainties, and should be tailored and specific to the patient's situation rather than a generic statement.

Insufficient evidence	Needs further development	Competent	Excellent
	Arranges definite appointments for follow up regardless of need or the nature of the problem.	Suggests a variety of follow-up arrangements that are safe and appropriate, whilst also enhancing patient autonomy.	Able to challenge unrealistic patient expectations and consulting patterns with regard to follow up of current and future problems.

Patient: *"It's reassuring to know I can talk to you about anything if I feel something isn't right, that is really so helpful to know."*

Mutually agreed.

Chapter 34

Mutual negotiation

The CSA assesses the doctor's ability to work in partnership with the patient to achieve the task of the consultation efficiently, reaching a mutually agreed plan in response to the preferences and concerns of the patient in a safe way.[1] The partnership is achieved through the doctor's willingness to encourage the patient's contribution at all stages of the consultation.[3] The doctor needs to recognise that the health decision being made is the patient's, and that their autonomy should be encouraged by providing them with information to help in making decisions. The best way to achieve a mutually agreed plan is for the doctor to gather information from the patient which allows the doctor to find a common ground for negotiation, and also offers options of treatment in a suggestive rather than a prescriptive manner, thereby giving the patient an opportunity to make decisions for themselves. This is different from asking the patient whether they agree with a decision already made by the doctor.

43-year-old man

Patient: *"Doctor, I have an itchy backside which has been a bit of a nuisance over the last few months. I have kept my piles under control with over-the-counter medication but it does flare up from time to time. I'm quite sure the irritation isn't due to the piles, and have seen one of your colleagues about that. When the piles flare up, they respond very well to the cream, but this irritation hasn't got any better despite getting through two tubes of the cream. I thought I'd get your opinion."*

The doctor allows the patient to tell their story, actively listens, seeking to understand the line of thought of the patient, and their reason for attending. The doctor should explore the patient's problems in such a way as to understand why they have attended and the nature of any likely decisions. The line of enquiry the doctor chooses should encourage the patient to share their experience of the problem and within that context develop an understanding of the patient's thoughts and perspectives.

Doctor: *"It sounds like you suspect something else might be causing this itching."*

Reflective statement to help reassure the patient that they have been heard, but also a good tool to encourage the patient to share their unique experience without interruptions from any doctor-centred questions. Paraphrasing is a useful reflective way to achieve this.

> *Positive CSA indicator*
> * Explores the patient's agenda, health beliefs and preferences.

Patient: *"I've been observing the area very carefully to see if I can identify any particular thing that causes the irritation. The only thing I've noticed is that the irritation is always worse* *towards the evening after work, and I'm not sure if it's due to how long we have to sit in one place at work. At the same time, I've also noticed that whenever I have my cereals in the morning with milk, I tend to get more irritation on those particular days. I know it sounds a bit weird but it certainly has been the case. I've stopped having milk, but unfortunately that hasn't stopped the irritation. I bought a cream different from my normal pile cream the last time it flared up, and it's also possible the new cream might have started off the irritation. I didn't want to keep guessing, so thought I would get it diagnosed properly."*

Patient is sharing their health beliefs. These are issues they have thought about and worked with trying the resolve the problem, and the information is important for the doctor to understand the reason why they have attended, and the nature of decision they have attended to make. They probably would like a diagnosis but also a clarification of the issue with milk and the cream for piles. This understanding focuses the consultation and improves the doctor's understanding of the patient experience, putting the problem in context.

> **Positive CSA indicator**
> * Clarifies the problem and nature of the decision required.

Doctor: *"I can see you've tried to work out the definite cause of the irritation."*

Clarifying the task and nature of the decision to be made.

Checking patient's understanding.

Patient: *"When I checked on the NHS website, it mentioned several conditions that can cause irritation in that area and one of the conditions – lichen sclerosis – sounded like exactly what I've been experiencing. It recommended seeing your doctor to discuss its treatment."*

The doctor clarifies the reason for attending, discovers the patient's concerns and expectations. The doctor understands the problem from the patient's perspective and their unique experience. The doctor understands what the main task is, and the focus of the consultation. This understanding is what the CSA assesses.

> **Positive CSA indicators**
> * Explores the patient's agenda, health beliefs and preferences.
> * Appears alert to verbal and non-verbal cues.

Doctor: *"Tell me a little about how the itching feels."*

This nature of questioning using an open question targeted at understanding the problem from the patient's experience of it will enable the doctor to recognise the likely cause of the condition presented, improving their focus for the rest of the data gathering. The severity and impact of a condition can also be appreciated from the patient's description of the problem by carefully observing verbal and non-verbal cues.

Patient: *"It's mostly OK in the mornings and I don't necessarily feel it every day, but the days when I feel the irritation it can be quite a nuisance. The only thing I find useful sometimes is a cold bath in the evening or a good moisturising cream. It's definitely much worse in the evenings after work, especially after a long day when it's been quite hot at work."*

Doctor gains an insight into the severity of the problem and the impact on the patient. Questions like "How bad has it been?" are useful in exploring the impact of a problem, improving the doctor's understanding of the patient's experience.

Positive CSA indicators
- Explores the impact of the illness on the patient's life.
- Elicits psychological and social information to place the patient's problem in context.

The doctor now uses closed questions to clarify the connection between the OTC cream and the itching. Clarifies the connection with the work situation and understands the working environment, clarifies the milk situation to help develop a functional solution if needed. The closed questions should show some logic in working out the most likely cause of the irritation using the information available to the doctor, but excluding red flags.

Positive CSA indicators
- Is appropriately selective in the choice of enquiries, examinations and investigations.
- Data gathering appears to be guided by the probabilities of disease.

Doctor: *"Is it OK if I have a look to help me understand the rash a little bit more?"*

Diagnosis: eczematous area around the perianal skin with no hardening or whitening. No typical features of lichen sclerosis. No piles.

Doctor: *"The area where you experience the itching does look a little inflamed, and I know you'd wondered about the possibility of lichen sclerosis, but I can't see the typical changes on the skin that we associate with the condition. You're right that it also causes a lot of itching in the area, just like you've experienced. It's often difficult to be entirely sure of the exact cause of this type of irritation, as no matter the cause it is likely the inflammation would have a similar appearance. It's possible the sweating at work may be making the situation worse, which would explain why you feel irritated more towards the end of the day. I wouldn't have expected milk to cause such a localised irritation."*

The doctor uses the explanation to respond to the patient's expectations, which in this case is the clarification of the cause of the irritation. The doctor recognises that for them to achieve a mutual agreement, they both have to share their thoughts and feelings about the situation, and then find a common ground to agree on a plan of action based on a shared understanding. The doctor uses their understanding of the patient's experience to find practical solutions to the patient's problem.

Positive CSA indicators
- Provides explanations that are relevant and understandable to the patient.
- Shows responsiveness to the patient's preferences, feelings and expectations.
- Enhances patient autonomy.

Insufficient evidence	Needs further development	Competent	Excellent
	Makes decisions by applying rules, plans or protocols.	Thinks flexibly around problems, generating functional solutions.	No longer relies on rules or protocols but is able to use and justify discretionary judgement in situations of uncertainty or complexity, for example in patients with multiple problems.

Doctor: *"Do you think perhaps it might be a good idea to avoid using the OTC cream for now to see if things improve, and we can use something else instead in the area if you notice the piles coming back?"*

Suggestive offer of management option.

> **Positive CSA indicator**
> - Is cooperative and inclusive in approach.

Patient: *"That's fine."*

Doctor: *"I wonder if there are things we could do to improve the situation at work?"*

> **Positive CSA indicators**
> - Works in partnership, finding common ground to develop a shared management plan.
> - Offers appropriate and feasible management options.

Patient: *"I'll speak to my boss about our chat to see if he would allow me to sit closer to the windows, and maybe think about wearing some looser cotton clothing."*

Doctor: *"I think whatever we can do to reduce the area being moist from sweating is likely to help the situation, and I think the idea of taking care with your choice of clothing is very reasonable. For the area that's inflamed already, there are a few things we can do to help the situation. Inflammations of the skin like this one respond well to creams containing steroids. I'm not sure whether you've heard of them or used any before. They're useful when used only for short periods of time to settle the inflammation, and I think it's likely to help resolve the irritation. I would normally expect the area to improve within a few days of applying the treatment, and if that happens then perhaps it would be advisable to continue the treatment for a period of 2 weeks. We can then have another look to make sure everything is resolving, but in the event that it doesn't make any difference or the irritation gets worse, then you must let me know. Although there are no features now suggesting anything else like lichen sclerosis, we can still reconsider perhaps investigating it further if the irritation does not resolve."*

> **Positive CSA indicators**
> - Makes plans that reflect the natural history of common problems.
> - Offers appropriate and feasible management options.
> - Uses an incremental approach, using time and accepting uncertainty.

Patient: *"OK."*

The negotiation should involve the doctor using their understanding of the patient's experience to offer options they consider feasible and appropriate for the specific patient's experience of the problem, in an incremental approach. The patient is given information regarding any of the possible options to help them to make the decision.

> **Positive CSA indicator**
> - Works in partnership, finding common ground to develop a shared management plan.

Chapter 35

Dealing with a discordant request

31-year-old man

Patient: *"I've had this cough for a whole 3 days now, and I'm wondering if you can prescribe a course of antibiotics to nip it in the bud."*

Active listening to understand the patient's request. Although the patient's reason for attending seems very obvious, the focus should be on developing a relationship with the patient to be able to work in partnership to decide on the best way to manage their problem. They have indicated a potential preference but have also attended to get clarification from the doctor, and this clarification is much easier for the patient to accept if their thoughts are explored and understood, so that the doctor is able to offer an explanation and advice that reflects a genuine understanding of the patient's own feelings, and the impact of the problem.

Doctor: *"Tell me what has happened exactly."*

Reflective question to understand the patient's experience and the description of the problem. The doctor chose this question as it is likely to be open enough to encourage the patient to share their experience and in that context the doctor gains insight into the nature of the problem, and builds a therapeutic relationship with the patient through understanding their perspective.

> *Positive CSA indicator*
> - Gathers information from history taking, examination and investigation in a systematic and efficient manner.

Patient: *"We've only just returned from holiday in Spain. The cough started on our last day, and has gradually worsened. I was hoping it would resolve on its own, but it has in fact got worse. I'm hoping to get on top of it quite quickly."*

Doctor gains an insight into the patient's request. Verbal cues, able to appreciate the context of the problem. The doctor continues to explore the patient's request as this will shed more light on their reason for attending and the nature of the decision they have attended to make.

Doctor: *"It sounds like it's bothered you quite a bit and you're keen to get it resolved quickly."*

Doctor explores the severity and impact on the patient, to place the problem in the context of the patient's experience.

Patient: *"We have a 2-month-old baby, so I'm trying everything I can not to transfer it to her. She is well but I know with babies that a chest infection can be fatal. My colleague at work lost their baby from a chest infection, although he was premature. That has bothered me a lot since the cough started. Normally I wouldn't have come in with just a cough."*

Patient's concerns. Reason for attending. Nature of the decision to be made. Discovering this information later in the consultation would not give doctor the same level of context, empathy and focus required to gather data and advise the patient appropriately. This is a common cause of discordance in the consultation. An assumption of the problem or a focus on the problem mainly from the onset is likely to lead to an argument about whether or not an antibiotic might be needed, especially if the doctor proceeds to find a normal throat and chest on examination. The approach followed above improves rapport, as the doctor develops a good empathetic relationship with the patient based on his understanding of their experience of the problem. The doctor is more likely to respond to this understanding when offering or not offering any treatment.

Doctor: *"I can understand why that would have made you consider early treatment. It sounds like you suspect antibiotics would resolve this particular episode."*

Clarifying patient's understanding. Preparing common ground for a shared decision, using their understanding of the nature of the decision the patient has attended to make.

Patient: *"I know antibiotics aren't helpful for colds, but it can be difficult to tell for sure whether it's a cold or a chest infection. I didn't want to gamble, so thought I would come along and get clarification from you, just to be on the safe side. I'm also starting a new job in the bank and didn't want to turn up on my first day with a nasty cough."*

Patient's health belief. The doctor uses this information when giving the patient his thoughts and finding a common ground.

Doctor: *"I'm glad you've come in to speak to me about it. I'd like to ask some specific questions to help me understand the chances of the cough being a cold or a chest infection."*

Reason for attending clarified.

The doctor uses focused questions to characterise the cough, specifically confirming the likely nature of the cause. Excludes red flags. Verifies other aspects of the history necessary to formulate the most likely aetiology. It may be necessary to verify the health of the baby and details about the birth, etc. The nature of enquiry is likely to focus on both clarifying the doctor's agenda and the patient's concerns.

Focused question targeted at the problem and the task based on the doctor's understanding of the patient's thoughts and experience. The doctor is expected to apply their knowledge of likelihood to focus their closed question enough to both clarify their suspicions and exclude any sinister features and address the patient's concerns.

Doctor: *"Is it OK for me to have a look at the throat and the chest for you?"*

Examination. Clear chest and normal throat but slightly inflamed. Temperature normal.

Diagnosis: URTI

Doctor: *"I've had a listen to your chest and examined your throat. I've also checked your temperature and felt around your neck. I would expect to hear noises in the chest if you had a chest infection, but the chest sounded very clear. The throat looks a little bit red but is showing no evidence of an infection that would require an antibiotic. Your temperature is also normal. You're right about how it can be difficult to differentiate a cold and a chest infection, but the examination finding can be very helpful in determining the presence of a chest infection. From the examination, it's more likely you've picked up a cold rather than a chest infection. Because antibiotics do not work on colds, the only thing we can do to prevent your cold from spreading to another person is to take precautions to prevent droplets from sneezing and ensure good hand hygiene."*

Giving explanation to respond to the understanding of the patient. Addressing patient's concerns. It is important to notice that the doctor did not use terms like virus and bacteria, responding to their understanding of the patient, which explains why the initial exploration should not be considered as just routine but at the heart of patient-centredness.

> **Positive CSA indicators**
> - Communicates risk effectively to patients.
> - Shows responsiveness to the patient's preferences, feelings and expectations.
> - Enhances patient autonomy.
> - Provides explanations that are relevant and understandable to the patient.

Patient: *"I'm glad it's not a chest infection. I would rather avoid antibiotics if they're not needed, to be honest."*

Mutual agreement based on patient's concerns being addressed. In this case, even if the patient still really wanted to try antibiotics, they may understand the doctor's decision not to prescribe them. They are more likely to accept that decision if they feel they have played a role in the decision making because the doctor has encouraged their contribution to the consultation.

Doctor: *"Normally I would expect this kind of infection to resolve on its own. It can take from a few days to perhaps 2 weeks, but drinking plenty of fluids and resting would help the body recover. If you notice that you start to cough more or bring up coloured phlegm or have a fever, you must let me know, as that may be an indication that the infection is changing."*

Safety nets. This is an opportunity for the doctor to demonstrate a further responsiveness to their understanding of the patient's concerns and perspectives, providing more reassurance, maintaining rapport.

Doctor: *"I know you were more concerned about the baby and your work. The best way to stop infection like this from spreading is to make sure the droplets are covered with a tissue and by maintaining good hand hygiene, but I'm not sure how you would prefer to proceed with the situation at work."*

Patient: *"I don't feel unwell in myself really, and I think as long as it's not gone into the chest, I would be able to go into work. But I will keep my hands washed and be careful about spreading the germs."*

Doctor: *"Perhaps you can let them know how you're feeling beforehand, just to forewarn them. If you feel more unwell, like we discussed, then you must let me know and we can reassess the situation."*

Patient: *"OK."*

Chapter 36

Reassuring patients

Patient: *"I woke up three mornings ago and noticed that my left eye had gone very red. It's not painful or anything, and my vision hasn't changed. I've been trying to figure out what could have happened, but was hoping it would all resolve on its own. It hasn't changed since then, so I thought maybe I might need some drops to put in it."*

Clarifying the reason for attending.

The doctor needs to understand the patient's thoughts and experience of the situation, even though the opening statement might make it seem obvious what the patient may have attended to discuss. The line of enquiry should be open, to encourage the patient to share their thoughts and feelings about the problem. It is within this context that the doctor's understanding of the nature of the clinical problem and the patient develops, to give the doctor an insight into the exact reasons for the patient's presentation.

Doctor: *"It must have been a bit of a puzzle for you?"*

Exploring the patient's thoughts and understanding of the problem. Reflective question to encourage the patient to share their thoughts.

Patient: *"Initially I was really worried. I know sometimes people can bleed in the white part of the eye, as one of my friends had a similar bleed. I thought that it would have resolved by now if it was the same thing as my friend had. It got me thinking when the redness didn't resolve after 2 days. I wasn't sure whether I had walked into a branch somewhere or something like that, but I can't think of anything that would have caused it. I've been sneezing quite a lot over the last week, but I'm not sure that could cause something as bad as this. I thought about the possibility of an infection, when the redness wasn't going away on the third day. I'm partially blind in the right eye already, and wouldn't want anything to go wrong in my good left eye. I rely on this eye for my driving, as I am the main carer of my wife who is disabled."*

Patient's perspective. Impact of the problem on the patient and others. The reason for attending. The nature of the decision to be made. Genuine empathy. The doctor is able to efficiently focus the consultation on the main task. They can work in partnership with the patient due to this understanding, finding a common ground. They can improve the explanation they offer to the patient using this understanding. They can address the main decision the patient has attended to make. The doctor keeps the patient safe using closed questions targeted to the problem and red flags.

Insufficient evidence	Needs further development	Competent	Excellent
	Develops a relationship with the patient, which works, but is focused on the problem rather than the patient.	Explores and responds to the patient's agenda, health beliefs and preferences. Elicits psychological and social information to place the patient's problem in context.	Incorporates the patient's perspective and context when negotiating the management plan.

Doctor: *"I can understand how that must have made you feel. I'd like to ask you some specific questions to be able to understand the problem a bit better."*

Doctor empathises more appropriately and gains more understanding of the patient's concerns and feelings.

The doctor uses closed questions to clarify the history of sneezes, exclude sign of infections or trauma. Excludes red flags; vision and pains. This is done using awareness of the prevalence of the potential causes of a common presentation, and completing the doctor's agenda, which is to exclude alternative causes. The focus is achieved from understanding and clarifying the nature of the experience of the problem by the patient.

Insufficient evidence	Needs further development	Competent	Excellent
	Accumulates information from the patient that is mainly relevant to their problem. Uses existing information in the patient records.	Systematically gathers information, using questions appropriately targeted to the problem without affecting patient safety. Understands the importance of, and makes appropriate use of, existing information about the problem and the patient's context.	Expertly identifies the nature and scope of enquiry needed to investigate the problem, or multiple problems, within a short time-frame. Prioritises problems in a way that enhances patient satisfaction.

Doctor: *"Is it OK if I have a look at the eye and check your blood pressure?"*

Examination: subconjunctival haemorrhage. BP 125/80 mmHg. VA normal.

The choice of examination should be focused on verifying the likely cause as suspected from the history and also addressing the patient's concerns, and in this case a visual acuity may help reassure the patient further. The choice of examination should be logical and focused.

Insufficient evidence	Needs further development	Competent	Excellent
	Chooses examination broadly in line with the patient's problem(s).	Chooses examinations appropriately targeted to the patient's problem(s).	Proficiently identifies and performs the scope of examination necessary to investigate the patient's problem(s).

Positive CSA indicator
- Data gathering appears to be guided by the probabilities of disease.

Doctor: *"It looks like a small vessel has burst in the white area of the eye, as you had suspected in the beginning. The appearance of the red area is typical of a burst small vessel in the white part of the eye. The fact that you don't have any pains and your vision hasn't changed is reassuring, and makes it unlikely to have been anything more serious. It's very possible that the episode of heavy sneezing and blowing your nose may have put a lot of pressure on the vessel. I would expect the redness to resolve on its own within a few days without causing any problems to your vision."*

Explanation of the problem using the understanding of the patient's perspective. Addressing the patient's concerns. Achieving the task of the consultation in partnership with the patient due to the recognition of the contribution of the patient to the consultation.

Positive CSA indicator
- Provides explanations that are relevant and understandable to the patient.

Insufficient evidence	Needs further development	Competent	Excellent
From the available evidence, the doctor's performance cannot be placed on a higher point of this developmental scale.	Provides explanations that are medically correct but doctor-centred.	Uses the patient's understanding to help improve the explanation offered.	Uses a variety of communication techniques and materials (e.g. written or electronic) to adapt explanations to the needs of the patient.

In this case this explanation addresses the patient's reason for attending, which isn't a diagnosis of the red eye, but to confirm whether it is a benign bleed, to exclude any vision-threatening problems, and verify whether the sneezing would have played a role. This consultation may provide an opportunity for the doctor to explore the sneezing problem further.

Doctor: *"Assuming you notice that your vision changes in any way or you start feeling any pains in that eye, please let me know as soon as you can so we can review the decision again, but it's very unlikely that will happen."*

Patient: *"Thanks."*

Chapter 37

Explaining a diagnosis using the patient's understanding

Patient: *"I've had this pain at the base of my left thumb for over 6 months. The other doctor arranged an X-ray, which showed only mild arthritis, but the pain has been unbearable at times despite all the creams I've been applying to it. I've come to get a referral to see someone for an injection."*

The doctor actively listens to the opening statement of the patient. The most important task at this stage is to develop an understanding of the patient's experience and not to focus mainly on the clinical problem. "Why they want an injection", "How bad the problem has been", "How it affects the patient", "What they have done about it so far", "What they understand or thought about the problem". Having these thoughts in the mind of the doctor will help them empathise more appropriately and enhances the choice of reflective question the doctor uses to encourage the patient to share their views, understanding, thoughts and experience. The patient's own views will help the doctor to focus the enquiries further in identifying both the nature of the problem and the tasks the patient has attended to resolve.

Doctor: *"I can see that this has really caused you a little bit of a problem. It sounds like you have considered an injection to the best option for you."*

Reflective question, showing willingness to encourage the patient's contribution.

Positive CSA indicators
- Explores the patient's agenda, health beliefs and preferences.
- Appears alert to verbal and non-verbal cues.
- Responds to needs and concerns with interest and understanding.

Patient: *"I think I've done everything I can to resolve it for now. I've been massaging the thumb with Deep Heat, and even rubbed in some hydrocortisone cream that I had in the cupboard from my previous visit. It's making life a bit difficult now, but I have a friend at the clubhouse who had huge success from an injection into her knee joint. She said the injection contained steroids, which magically resolved the arthritis, which is why I tried the steroid cream before booking this appointment. I've never had a joint injection before, so I can't say that I'm totally convinced of its safety. I don't know what you think?"*

Patient's understanding. Health beliefs. Preference. Reason for attending. The doctor is able to focus the consultation to achieve the task, responding to the patient's perspective, by focusing their approach mainly on developing a relationship with the patient.

Insufficient evidence	Needs further development	Competent	Excellent
	Develops a relationship with the patient, which works, but is focused on the problem rather than the patient.	Explores and responds to the patient's agenda, health beliefs and preferences. Elicits psychological and social information to place the patient's problem in context.	Incorporates the patient's perspective and context when negotiating the management plan.

Doctor: *"We will discuss the steroids later, but it sounds like this problem has really affected you a lot."*

Impact on the patient and context.

> **Positive CSA indicators**
> - Explores the impact of the illness on the patient's life.
> - Elicits psychological and social information to place the patient's problem in context.

Patient: *"The doctor did say nothing will really reverse the arthritis, but it's the pain that bothers me most. I'm beginning to struggle to hold the golf club, and I'm one of the leading team members at my local club. Even opening cans of food can be a little difficult, as I'm left-handed. I really don't know exactly what the injection does, but am really happy to discuss any alternative."*

Patient's thoughts and preference, the impact of the problem. The doctor puts the problem in the patient's context and gains more insight into the reason for attending.

The doctor is able to focus the data gathering from this point to not only confirm the nature of the clinical problem, but also to address the patient's agenda. This approach, if learned, prevents the doctor from using formulaic questions in understanding the patient's experience, shifting the focus from the disease to the patient's experience of the disease. This focus on the patient's experience is what is assessed in the CSA.

The doctor uses closed questions to confirm the diagnosis. Excludes red flags; other joints.

Drug history. PMH.

Doctor: *"Is it OK if I have a look at the hands?"*

Examination: mild tenderness CMC joint. No inflammation.

Diagnosis: mild CMC joint OA.

Doctor: *"The pain you're experiencing is from the joint at the base of the thumb, and you're right that it is probably due to the arthritis. I know you've been doing all you can to help resolve the pain. Steroid injections can help reduce the pain, and are usually effective but not always. The effect of the relief can vary as well. Sometimes patients can be pain-free for a period of a few months to years, and it's difficult to determine who will benefit for longer. I know you would prefer to go for this option, but I'm not sure whether you've considered other non-invasive ways that we can control the pain. The injection doesn't reverse the arthritis, like you've said, but can help keep the pain under control. Although they're usually* *safe, every joint injection can have potential complications like infections afterwards, or occasionally the pains may get worse after an injection."*

Doctor shares their thoughts, showing responsiveness to their understanding of the nature of the decision the patient has attended to make. The doctor uses their understanding of the patient's ideas to improve the explanation they offer, addressing the patient's agenda. The explanation focuses on the main reason the patient has attended. The information was given in a way to reflect an understanding of the fact that the patient was considering mainly pain relief and understood that the injection does not cure the problem.

> *Positive CSA indicators*
> - Shows responsiveness to the patient's preferences, feelings and expectations.
> - Enhances patient autonomy.
> - Provides explanations that are relevant and understandable to the patient.

Doctor: *"I know you've tried Deep Heat and hydrocortisone. Hydrocortisone applied on the skin wouldn't normally get deep enough to help the joints, which is why we don't normally recommend it for joint pains. I'm not sure whether you've considered perhaps using a non-steroidal anti-inflammatory cream instead of the Deep Heat to see if you would benefit from that?"*

Suggesting options. Seeking common ground. The approach encourages further patient contribution. Occasionally some important aspects of the patient's perspective can become apparent during the decision-making stages.

> *Positive CSA indicators*
> - Makes plans that reflect the natural history of common problems.
> - Offers appropriate and feasible management options.

Patient: *"I didn't know you could get anti-inflammatory medication in creams. It sounds like a good idea, and I'd like to give that a go first, because as you said the injection really should be a last resort."*

Mutually accepted.

> *Positive CSA indicator*
> - Works in partnership, finding common ground to develop a shared management plan.

Doctor: *"Perhaps you could combine that with taking some paracetamol, if you don't get much benefit from using the cream on its own."*

Incremental approach of offering options. Seeking common ground and mutual agreement.

> *Positive CSA indicator*
> - Uses an incremental approach, using time and accepting uncertainty.

Doctor: *"I know you get into difficulty when you use the thumb for doing things at home, but it's often beneficial to keep exercising the joint from time to time. I'll give you a guide that will help you with how and when to do these exercises to keep the joint from feeling stiff and more painful to use."*

Health promotion.

> **Positive CSA indicator**
> - Encourages improvement, rehabilitation and, where appropriate, recovery.

Doctor: *"Perhaps we can see how you get on with these strategies, and we can consider other options if you don't get any benefit. If it gets to a point where you find that you are no longer able to cope with the pains, you can come back in and we could go through other options."*

Safety net, using incremental approach.

> **Positive CSA indicator**
> - Uses an incremental approach, using time and accepting uncertainty.

Patient: *"Absolutely. I will let you know how I get on."*

Decision made together.

Chapter 38

Checking the patient's understanding

It is important for the doctor to establish the patient's views and thoughts before discussing the treatment options, so that they can offer their thoughts to the patient using a language that takes into account their understanding of the patient's experience. This will then enhance the patient's autonomy by improving their understanding of the choices offered. This reduces the chances of an occurrence of discordance during the decision-making stages of the consultation.[5] The doctor should foresee the nature of the conversation to be held in the decision-making, using their understanding of the patient's reasons for attending and knowledge of the natural courses of diseases. It is more effective for the doctor to develop understanding of the patient's experience by using an approach that encourages the patient to participate in the consultation both during the data gathering, by sharing their thoughts, and during the decision-making stages, by giving the patient opinions and being suggestive rather than instructive in their approach. The treatment options offered should reflect the doctor's understanding of the patient rather than being a list of all the possible treatment options of management of the particular clinical condition.

73-year-old man

Patient: *"I've come along today to get your opinion about these pains I've been getting in the small joint on the end of my finger. The area has been a little prominent for the last few months but occasionally it gives me quite a lot of discomfort. I don't really know what the swelling is or what to do."*

The doctor listens actively to gain an understanding of what exactly the patient has said. Paying close attention to the line of thought of the patient, to understand the reason for attending and the nature of the decision the patient has attended to make. The approach should be to consider reflective questions that focus on understanding the reason for the patient's visit, and to clarify the task ahead. This is also a good opportunity to screen for other problems, etc. The temptation is to rush in to get the chronology of the story, which will help the doctor make a diagnosis. The diagnosis of the problem is expected to be made through the doctor's recognition of a common condition in general practice.

Sometimes doctors use generic questions to encourage the patient to continue talking, such as "Tell me how it all started". If they are used without actively listening or out of context, they may be perceived by the patient as illogical. It is rewarding to use questions that demonstrate a genuine understanding of what the patient has said to make the patient feel heard, improving rapport and encouraging further contribution from the patient. Reflective questions that are empathetic can be very effective.

Doctor: *"It sounds like you are now really struggling with the pains. Did you have any thoughts as to why they may have become worse?"*

Reflective question to explore the patient's understanding and experience of the problem. The nature of the question demonstrates the doctor's understanding of what the patient has said and may be thinking about.

Insufficient evidence	Needs further development	Competent	Excellent
	Accumulates information from the patient that is mainly relevant to their problem. Uses existing information in the patient records.	Systematically gathers information, using questions appropriately targeted to the problem without affecting patient safety. Understands the importance of, and makes appropriate use of, existing information about the problem and the patient's context.	Expertly identifies the nature and scope of enquiry needed to investigate the problem, or multiple problems, within a short time-frame. Prioritises problems in a way that enhances patient satisfaction.

Patient: *"I had gout in my toes a few years ago. I was still working then, but it normally always resolved with simple painkillers. The doctor at the time suggested some medicines to take regularly, but I declined going down that route at the time, as I felt perhaps it wasn't happening too often. I haven't really had any problems with gout since then – until now. I've now retired and have a lot of time to myself to do things, and my lifestyle hasn't changed really, apart from being put on blood pressure medication recently. I wasn't sure whether these tablets might have anything to do with the gout coming back."*

The doctor understands the patient's thoughts about the problem, and the nature of the reason for the patient's attendance. The uniqueness of the patient's experience of the problem is important. This understanding will focus the consultation to the task. The patient's concerns regarding the new medication should be taken note of. The best way to achieve this understanding is to genuinely show interest in the patient's problem and focus the initial attention to understand the patient in a holistic way.

Doctor: *"It sounds like you would like to verify the cause of the changes in the finger and what to do about them."*

Reflective question to clarify the patient's reason for attending.

Patient: *"I'd really like to confirm if it is indeed gout, and maybe discuss going on those preventive medications if you think it's necessary."*

Patient's expectations. Once the tasks are clarified the doctor has an idea of the direction the consultation should follow in response to the unique characteristics of that patient, bearing in mind that the doctor's agenda will need to be completed using closed questions to focus the data gathering to reflect the insight the doctor has gained.

Doctor: *"What are you doing to help the pains now?"*

Patient: *"I don't really need to take any painkillers as most of the time it isn't too bad. It can be a little tricky when I open cans at home, but I've bought a new can opener which has solved that problem for me."*

> **Positive CSA indicator**
> - Explores the impact of the illness on the patient's life.

Signposting. The doctor clarifies the nature of the joint problem, excludes red flags, using closed questions to exclude other possibilities, etc. They are now more likely to also focus on the patient's lifestyle and understanding previous episodes of the problem and what investigations have been done.

Doctor: *"Is it OK if I examine the hand?"*

Examination: mild distal osteoarthritis.

Doctor: *"I've had a look. I can see the area around the end of the finger that is prominent. The appearance is not what I would expect from gout. Gout often causes a lot of redness and swelling, but in this case there are mostly bony prominences and no redness around the joint. It looks like changes that are typical of wear and tear in the small joint of the finger. I don't think it's anything to do with the tablets as the changes are more like those that would have happened gradually over a long time."*

Doctor uses the explanation to respond to their understanding of the patient's thoughts and health beliefs. Explanations offered in this way are more likely to be understood by the patient, and directly address both their concerns and the reason for attending. The doctor achieves the task of the consultation, responding to their understanding of the patient's views.

> **Positive CSA indicator**
> - Provides explanations that are relevant and understandable to the patient.

Insufficient evidence	Needs further development	Competent	Excellent
	Uses a rigid or formulaic approach to achieve the main tasks of the consultation.	Achieves the tasks of the consultation, responding to the preferences of the patient in an efficient manner.	Appropriately uses advanced consultation skills, such as confrontation or catharsis, to achieve better patient outcomes.

Patient: *"I thought so, because it doesn't quite feel as bad as the pains I had a few years ago, when the doctor diagnosed gout. I'm glad I don't have to go on regular medication."*

Task achieved but done in partnership with the patient, as their views and contribution have been taken into account in the decision-making.

Doctor: *"I know you're coping well without any painkillers, but I'm not sure whether you've perhaps considered anything else that might help relieve the pains, like gentle exercises of the hands?"*

Insufficient evidence	Needs further development	Competent	Excellent
	Communicates management plans but without negotiating with, or involving, the patient.	Works in partnership with the patient, negotiating a mutually acceptable plan that respects the patient's agenda and preference for involvement.	Whenever possible, adopts plans that respect the patient's autonomy. When there is a difference of opinion the patient's autonomy is respected and a positive relationship is maintained.

Patient: *"Anything that can help apart from tablets."*

Doctor: *"Doing gentle exercises helps to keep the small joint moving and stops it from getting stiff and more difficult to move. If it helps, I could give you some information on some of these exercises to try."*

> *Positive CSA indicators*
> - Encourages improvement, rehabilitation and, where appropriate, recovery.
> - Encourages the patient to participate in appropriate health promotion and disease prevention strategies.

Patient: *"I will certainly give that a go."*

Doctor: *"I wouldn't expect any sudden changes in the situation, but assuming you do notice any sudden change in the pains or redness, you must let me know."*

Managing patient's concerns and the uncertainties.

To achieve the competency levels assessed in the CSA, the doctor should be fluent in using communication skills to encourage the patient to contribute their thoughts, feelings, concerns, expectations, preferences and experience of the problem not simply as a part of history taking but as the **focus** of the data gathering and the management of their condition.

References

1. Royal College of General Practitioners MRCGP Clinical Skills Assessment. Available at: www.rcgp.org.uk/training-exams/mrcgp-exams-overview/mrcgp-clinical-skills-assessment-csa.aspx (accessed 31 March 2017).

2. The Training & Development World. Available at: http://thetrainingworld.com/faq/roledisad.htm (accessed 31 March 2017).

3. Lee GV and Barnett BG (1994). Using reflective questioning to promote collaborative dialogue. *Journal of Staff Development* 15:16. Available at: https://learningforward.org/docs/jsd/lee151.pdf?sfvrsn=0 (accessed 31 March 2017).

4. Revisiting Models of the Consultation. Available at: www.essentialgptrainingbook.com/resources/web_chapter_04/04%20consultation%20models.pdf (accessed 31 March 2017).

5. Fassaert T, van Dulmen S, Schellevis F, and Bensing J (2007). Active listening in medical consultations: development of the Active Listening Observation Scale (ALOS-global). *Patient Education and Counselling* 68:258. Available at: www.ncbi.nlm.nih.gov/pubmed/17689042 (accessed 31 March 2017).